Postpartum Depression

TCS MENTAL HEALTH

Postpartum Depression

A guide for front-line health and social service providers

Lori E. Ross, PhD

Cindy-Lee Dennis, RN, PhD

Emma Robertson Blackmore, PhD

Donna E. Stewart, MD, FRCPC

Writing and Editing Assistance
by June Engel, PhD

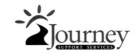
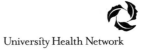
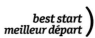

Library and Archives Canada Cataloguing in Publication
Postpartum depression: a guide for front line health and social service providers/Lori E. Ross ... [et al.].
Includes bibliographical references and index.
ISBN 0-88868-485-1
1. Postpartum depression. I. Ross, Lori Elizabeth, 1976-
11. Centre for Addiction and Mental Health.
RG852.P66 2005   618.7'6
C2004-906916-0
Product Code P5600
Printed in Canada

For information on other Centre for Addiction and Mental Health publications or to place an order, please contact:
Marketing and Sales Services
Centre for Addiction and Mental Health
33 Russell Street
Toronto, ON M5S 2S1
Canada
Tel.: 1 800 661-1111 or 416 595-6059 in Toronto
E-mail: marketing@camh.net
Website: www.camh.net

This book was produced by the following:
DEVELOPMENT: Julia Greenbaum, CAMH
EDITORIAL: Diana Ballon, CAMH; June Engel; Sharon Kirsch; Kelly Lamorie and Megan MacDonald
DESIGN: Mara Korkola, MFA, CAMH
PRINT PRODUCTION: Christine Harris, CAPPM, CAMH
MARKETING: Rosalicia Rondon, CAMH
TYPESETTER: Philip Sung Design Associates, Inc.

Disclaimer:
This publication makes every attempt to provide accurate and authoritative information in regard to the subject matter covered. It is sold with the understanding that the publisher is not engaged in rendering medical, psychological, social, financial, legal or other professional services. The contents of this publication are based on information available at the time of publication. However, in view of the possibility of human error or changes in medical science or relevant legislation, neither the authors, editors, publishers nor any other party who has been involved in the preparation of this publication warrant that the information is in every respect accurate or complete, and they are not responsible for any errors or omissions or for the results obtained for the use of such information. If expert assistance is needed, the services of a competent professional should be sought.

P5600/2897/02-05

Table of Contents

Acknowledgments

PARTNERING ORGANIZATIONS INVOLVED IN PROJECT PLANNING AND DRAFT
REVIEW PROCESSES

Best Start Resource Centre
Journey Support Services
Toronto Public Health
University Health Network, Women's Health Program

CAMH PROJECT MANAGER

Julia Greenbaum, MA

ASSISTANCE WITH WRITING AND DEVELOPMENTAL EDITING

June Engel, PhD, biochemist, medical author

Much gratitude is extended to the following reviewers for providing helpful feedback on earlier versions of this book and/or on specific sections or chapters:

SCIENTIFIC REVIEWER

Meir Steiner, MD, PhD, FRCPC,

Professor of Psychiatry & Behavioural Neurosciences and Obstetrics & Gynecology, McMaster University

Director, Women's Health Concerns Clinic, St. Joseph's Healthcare, Hamilton, Ontario

OTHER CONTENT REVIEWERS

Branka Agic, M.H.Sc., Community Health and Education Specialist, Centre for Addiction and Mental Health, Toronto, Ontario

Dawinder Bansal, RN, IBCLC, LCCE, Babies Best Start (Home Visiting Program), Home Visitor Supervisor, Toronto, Ontario

Saleha Bismilla, RN, BScN, Brampton, Ontario

Mara Celmins, RN, BScN, Health Promotion Consultant, Best Start Resource Centre, Toronto, Ontario

Gloria Chaim, MSW, RSW, Pathways to Healthy Families, Jean Tweed Centre, Toronto, Ontario

Rean Cross, Lucina Birth Services, Toronto, Ontario

Maureen Devolin, RN, BScN, Educator and Quality Improvement Specialist, Calgary Health Region, Calgary, Alberta

Dianne Edwards, BScN, Health Promoter, West Hill Community Services, Scarborough, Ontario

Donna Elliot, RN, BScN, IBCLC, Public Health Nurse, Leeds, Grenville and Lanark District Health Unit, Almonte, Ontario

Margaret Fairman, RN, BN, Women's Health Concerns Clinic, St. Joseph's Healthcare, Hamilton, Ontario

Sylvie Guenther, BSW, Centre for Addiction and Mental Health, Timmins, Ontario

Sepali Guruge, RN, BScN, M.Sc., PhD(c), Faculty of Nursing, University of Toronto, Toronto, Ontario

Denise Hébert, BScN, Family Health Specialist, Healthy Babies Healthy Children Program, Ottawa Public Health, Ottawa, Ontario

Sarafina Hui, BA, Community Health Promoter, The Scarborough Hospital - Family Wellness Centre, Scarborough, Ontario

Karen Jansen, MSW, RSW, Women's Health Concerns Clinic, St. Joseph's Healthcare, Hamilton, Ontario

Lise-Anne LaBelle,* RN (S.A.N.E.), Sexual Assault/Domestic Violence Treatment Program, Niagara Health System, St. Catharines, Ontario

Marian Law, MA, RD, Public Health Nutritionist, Toronto Public Health, Toronto, Ontario

Christine Long, BA, Journey Support Services, Mississauga, Ontario

Grazyna Mancewicz, RSW, M.Ed., Maternal Support Program, St. Joseph's Women's Health Centre, Toronto, Ontario

Teddy (Priscilla) McLaren, Aboriginal Healing and Wellness Coordinator, Nishnawbe-Gamik Friendship Centre, Sioux Lookout, Ontario

Linda McLean, C.Psych., Psychosocial Oncology & Palliative Care, Princess Margaret Hospital, Toronto, Ontario

Wendy Palermo, Survivor and Co-facilitator of support group, Welland, Ontario

Sandi Partridge, BA, BSW, RSW, Project Consultant, Centre for Addiction and Mental Health, Durham Region, Ontario

Nancy Poole, MA, Research Consultant on Women and Substance Use, B.C. Women's Hospital and British Columbia Centre of Excellence for Women's Health, Vancouver, British Columbia

Pat Ripmeester RN, BScN, IBCLC, Coordinator, Health Promotion & Clinical Services, Renfrew County & District Health Unit, Pembroke, Ontario

Kerri Ritchie, PhD, C.Psych., Department of Psychology and Maternal Fetal Medicine, The Ottawa Hospital, Ottawa, Ontario

K. Christine Sheeler, RN, Ottawa Hospital, Maternal – Newborn Care, Ottawa, Ontario

Jules E. Smith, MA, RCC, Provincial Reproductive Mental Health Program, B.C. Women's Hospital & Health Centre, Vancouver, British Columbia

Toronto Public Health Postpartum Depression Advisory Committee

Joan Turner, B.Ed., CCFE, Yukon Family Services Association, Whitehorse, Yukon

Bill Watson, MD, Family Physician, St. Michael's Hospital, Toronto, Ontario

Honey Watts, MA, RSW, Consultant and Project Coordinator, Calgary Health Region, 3 Cheers PPD Project, Calgary, Alberta

* *Sadly Lise-Anne Labelle died prior to this book's publication.*

THANKS ALSO GO TO THE FOLLOWING CAMH STAFF AND STUDENTS WHO PROVIDED RESEARCH AND DEVELOPMENT ASSISTANCE TO THE AUTHORS:

Patricia Donoghue
Amina Jabbar
Lana Mamisachvili

THE FOLLOWING PEOPLE CONTRIBUTED TO *POSTPARTUM DEPRESSION: LITERATURE REVIEW OF RISK FACTORS AND INTERVENTIONS*, COMMISSIONED BY TORONTO PUBLIC HEALTH, WHICH WAS A SOURCE FOR MANY EVIDENCE-BASED FINDINGS USED IN OUR BOOK:

Project leader
Donna E. Stewart, MD, FRCPC

Investigators
Cindy-Lee Dennis RN, PhD
Sherry Grace, PhD
Emma Robertson Blackmore, PhD
Tamara Wallington, MD, FRCPC

Assistants
Nalan Celasun, PhD
Danielle Rolfe, BPHE
Shephanie Sansom, MA

Lori Ross is grateful for the support of the Women's Mental Health and Addiction Research Section of CAMH for granting her time to work on this project.

We would also like to thank the many people who responded to our needs assessment questionnaire and provided us with useful suggestions and information that we used in the planning and development of the book.

A final thanks to Roxanne and Sheri who shared their personal stories for the sake of our book, and to the other women who submitted stories that, in the end, we were not able to include.

About the Authors

The four authors who have collaborated to produce *Postpartum Depression: A Guide for Front-Line Health and Social Service Providers* bring to it a wealth and unique blend of experience and expertise from wide-ranging fields of interest.

Lori Ross is a researcher whose main interests are in mental health issues during pregnancy and the postpartum period, particularly among marginalized populations. She is also a scientist at Toronto's Centre for Addiction and Mental Health (CAMH) and lead investigator on research projects examining mental health problems in immigrant mothers and in co-parenting lesbian and bisexual women.

Cindy-Lee Dennis is an assistant professor at the faculty of nursing, University of Toronto and the recipient of a Canadian Institutes of Health Research (CIHR) New Investigator Award. She has published numerous papers and conducted several evidence-based reviews and research studies on the detection, prevention and treatment of postpartum depression (PPD), including a recently published Cochrane systematic review and meta-analysis. She is currently the principal investigator of a large randomized controlled trial that is evaluating the effect of peer (mother-to-mother) support on the prevention of PPD and the effectiveness of screening procedures. The trial will also provide a complete economic evaluation.

Emma Robertson Blackmore is a psychologist who has spent the past 10 years in the United Kingdom working in clinical and academic settings with women with severe mental illness. Her special expertise is researching clinical and genetic aspects of puerperal psychosis and examining evidence-based risk factors for PPD. Dr. Robertson Blackmore completed post-doctoral fellowships at the University of Birmingham, England, and in the women's health program of the University Health Network, researching women and postpartum mood disorders. She has recently been appointed to the faculty in the department of psychiatry, University of Rochester Medical Center, New York, where she will be specializing in perinatal psychiatry.

Donna Stewart, professor and chair of women's health at the University Health Network and the University of Toronto, has 30 years of experience as a psychiatrist in the treatment, education and research of women's mental health problems, with a special focus on PPD. Dr. Stewart is the editor of four books on women's mental health and more than 200 peer-reviewed scientific papers and chapters, many of which have been translated for international use. She is a senior scientist at Toronto General Research Institute, president of the International Association of Women's Mental Health, and chair of the Section of Women's Mental Health for the World Psychiatric Association.

Introduction

Postpartum depression (PPD) is increasingly recognized as a serious, yet common, mental health issue for women. Unfortunately, much of this recognition has come from media attention associated with tragic cases of women with severe illnesses who, for one reason or another, did not receive the care they needed. These cases are not representative of most women who receive effective treatment and fully recover from PPD. Yet despite good reason for optimism, our sense is that many service providers feel unprepared to effectively address this significant health issue.

The first step in developing this resource was to survey front-line health and social service providers across Ontario to determine whether or not they needed a PPD resource, and if so, what kind of resource that would be. The overwhelming message we received was "yes": respondents indicated a clear need for a resource that would be relevant to Canadian service providers and one that would integrate the most current research into practical recommendations.

Encouraged by this enthusiastic response from potential users of our book, we invited Best Start, Journey Support Services, the University Health Network and Toronto Public Health to collaborate with us to develop a guide that would meet the needs of service providers. We hope that this book achieves our goal of creating a practical resource that translates PPD research into a format that a Canadian audience will find useful.

Many of the evidence-based findings and recommendations in this book draw on a report released late in 2003, entitled *Postpartum Depression: Literature Review of Risk Factors and Interventions*. This multi-authored, evidence-based review of PPD, prepared under the leadership of Dr. Donna Stewart, with funding from Toronto Public Health, contains contributions from two of our authors, Drs. Cindy-Lee Dennis and Emma Robertson Blackmore.

In several chapters of our book, we have tried to distill some of the scientific information from the literature review into an easy-to-understand reference guide format. For those who would like to learn more about the details of the research studies upon which we've made the evidence-based recommendations, we refer you to the Toronto Public Health report for a more in-depth discussion. You can access this report through the Toronto Public Health website at www.toronto.ca/health.

Our team of authors brings together expertise in psychology, psychiatry, nursing and research. These varied backgrounds have led us to take a *biopsychosocial* approach to PPD, which you will see integrated throughout the book. To us, taking a biopsychosocial approach means that we appreciate the important contributions of each woman's biological, psychological and social worlds to her postpartum experiences. We have found that understanding a new mother's mental health within her social context is key to providing her with helpful postpartum care, and we suggest ways of accomplishing this in our guide.

PPD research is a quickly growing field, yet to date researchers have conducted relatively few well-designed studies to answer important questions about screening, prevention and treatment. To address this gap, we have supplemented our evidence-based recommendations with recommendations based on our own and our colleagues' clinical experiences working with women with PPD. We have made every effort in this book to delineate which of our recommendations are evidence-based and which are practice-based, so that readers can make informed decisions about which strategies to incorporate into their own work.

1

Clinical Overview

What is postpartum depression? Does it differ from depression that occurs at other times?

How common is it?

What are its symptoms? How do clinicians diagnose it?

Once a woman has experienced postpartum depression, what are her chances of experiencing further episodes of depression?

What other types of mood disorders are common to the postpartum period?

Childbirth is a time of great physiological, psychological and social change. Having a psychiatric illness at such a crucial time in family life affects the mother, her partner, her children and family, and as such represents a considerable public health problem.

For centuries, medical professionals have noted the association between childbirth and mental illness. Studies have shown that women are at increased risk of developing a severe mood (or affective) disorder in the postpartum period, and are at a much greater risk of being admitted to a psychiatric hospital in the first month postpartum than at any other time in life (Kendell et al., 1987; Paffenbarger, 1982). Service providers working with new mothers will likely provide care to women who have the illness.

This chapter describes the affective states that are common following childbirth, focusing on **postpartum depression (PPD);** other disorders described include the baby blues and pinks, postpartum anxiety and **psychosis**. The chapter will differentiate between the disorders, and highlight problems and symptoms that may require intervention.

Postpartum Depression (PPD)

WHAT IS PPD?

Clinicians and researchers use the term "postpartum depression," or "PPD," to refer to non-psychotic depression that occurs shortly after childbirth.

DOES IT DIFFER FROM OTHER DEPRESSIONS?

Apart from the fact that it happens soon after childbirth, PPD is clinically no different from a depressive episode that occurs at any other time in a woman's life. The symptoms are the same as in general depression, and must meet the same criteria for diagnosis. However, not surprisingly, the content of the symptoms of PPD often focuses on motherhood or infant care topics.

WHAT CAUSES IT?

Although health professionals do not know what causes depression (and therefore PPD), they accept that there is no single cause. Physical, hormonal, social, psychological and emotional factors may all play a part in triggering the illness. This is known as the **biopsychosocial model** of depression, and is accepted by most researchers and clinicians. The factor or group of factors that trigger PPD vary from one individual to the other.

HOW COMMON IS IT?

PPD is the most common complication of child-bearing. Although the rates given in individual studies vary greatly, a meta-analysis of 59 studies of more than 12,000 women found that PPD affects an average of 13 per cent of women (O'Hara & Swain, 1996).

WHEN DOES IT START?

The time period used to define "postpartum" varies, from immediately following childbirth to four weeks (according to formal diagnostic classification systems) after childbirth or up to a year, according to some research studies. Symptoms usually begin within the first four weeks postpartum, although they can start up to 12 months afterwards. However, service providers may not detect and treat PPD until much later. Often, questioning will reveal that the symptoms actually began much earlier than the woman had disclosed to a health care provider.

HOW DO CLINICIANS DIAGNOSE IT?

A physician or licensed **psychologist** makes a formal diagnosis of depression. Professionals use numerous methods to elicit the information needed to make a diagnosis, including standardized clinical interviews. The clinician's judgment is essential in deciding whether or not an individual's symptoms meet diagnostic criteria, in terms of severity or duration of symptoms. The formal classification system used in North America is the American Psychiatric Association (APA) *Diagnostic and Statistical Manual of Mental Disorders, Fourth edition,* or *DSM-IV* (American Psychiatric Association, 1994). (See Figure 1–1 for *DSM-IV* criteria for a major depressive episode.)

To indicate an episode of PPD using *DSM-IV* criteria, the physician or psychologist would indicate that it is an episode of major depressive disorder with the specifier "postpartum onset" (which means that the symptoms occurred within four weeks of the woman's having given birth).

FIGURE 1–1

DSM-IV Symptoms of Major Depressive Disorder

Depressed Mood
Low, sad, empty
Irritable, restless
Tearful, crying more than usual
Feelings of inadequacy/being a bad mother
Excessive worry about baby's health or
generalized anxiety

Loss of Interest/Pleasure
Loss of interest in activities that would
usually bring pleasure
(e.g., being with baby; watching favourite
television show; reading; spending time
with partner, family or friends)

Two Weeks or More

Changes in Weight/Appetite
Weight gain or loss difficult to assess in new moms
Loss of desire for food, or lack of enjoyment of food

Sleep Disturbance
Difficulty falling asleep, difficulty waking, difficulty
staying asleep, inability to sleep when tired, inability
to fall back asleep after feeding

Physical Retardation or Agitation
Physical feelings of being slowed down (retardation)
or restless, being jumpy or on edge (agitation)

Fatigue
Feelings of tiredness persist, even after rest or sleep

Decreased Concentration or Ability to Think
"Slowed" thinking, difficulty concentrating on tasks
or ideas, inability to complete a task, difficulty
making decisions

Recurrent Thoughts of Death or Suicide
Thoughts that oneself or one's baby "would be
better off dead," or "the world is such an awful place
that we're better out of it"

Worthlessness/Guilt
Unrealistic, negative thoughts about one's worth
and feelings of excessive guilt over minor incidents
Feeling guilty about being ill is not sufficient for
a diagnosis

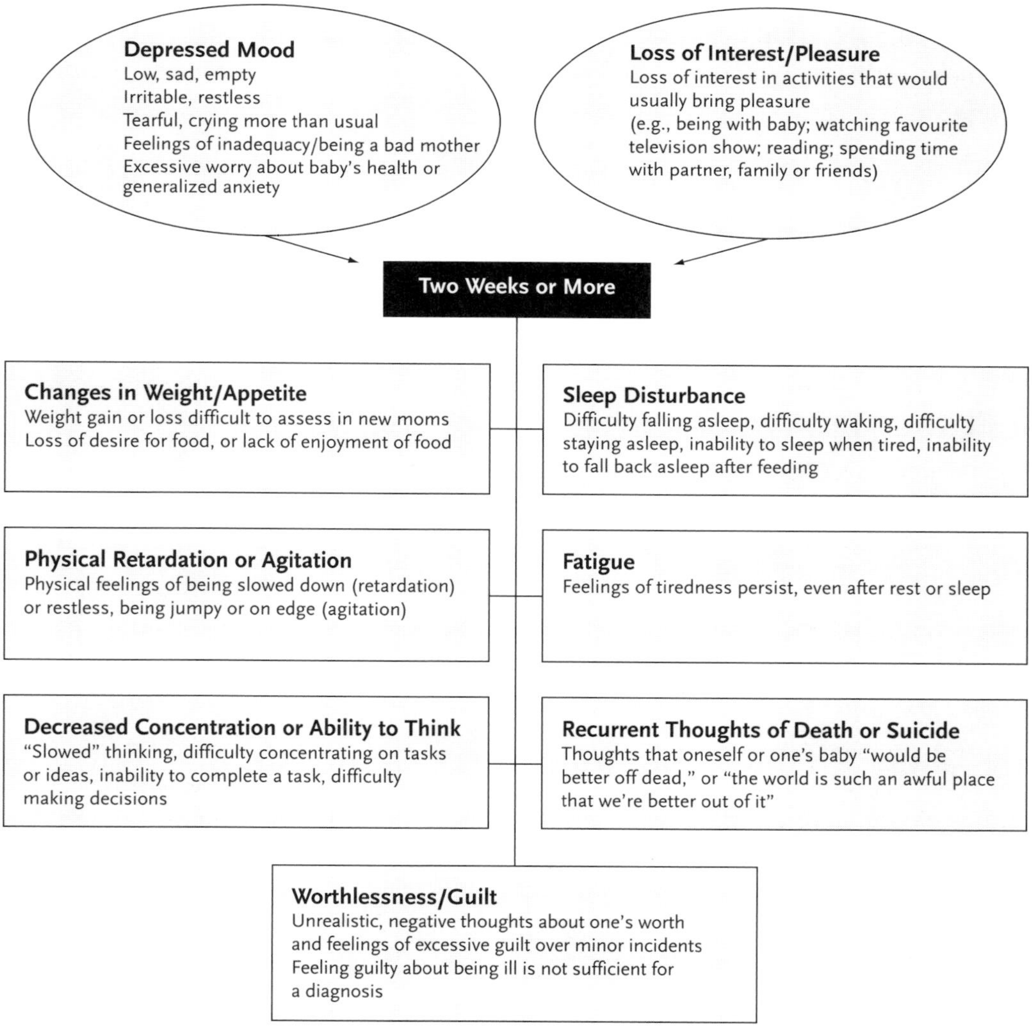

Adapted with permission from the *Diagnostic and Statistical Manual of Mental Disorders*, copyright 2000. American Psychiatric Association.

Individuals must have exhibited *either* a *depressed mood* or a *loss of interest or pleasure* in usual activities (called **anhedonia**) continually, for a minimum of two weeks. In addition, they must have experienced other symptoms from a given list of seven, for a minimum of two weeks.

A clinician will diagnose major depression if the individual has a low mood or anhedonia, plus four other symptoms (for a minimum of five symptoms). People with a low mood or anhedonia with fewer than four symptoms will receive a diagnosis of minor or moderate depression.

HOW CAN SERVICE PROVIDERS RULE OUT OTHER CAUSES?

It is imperative that the symptoms displayed a) represent a change from the individual's normal functioning and b) cause impairment in everyday life. Through referral to the family doctor or another physician, as appropriate, providers should rule out other medical conditions that may cause similar symptoms and may be common in the postpartum period (e.g., thyroid dysfunction, diabetes, anemia, autoimmune diseases).

HOW LONG DOES IT LAST?

The length of an episode varies from a number of weeks to a number of months. Some women say it can take up to a year for them to feel back to their normal selves. In a small number of cases, the episode may not remit and the women experience chronic episodes of depression.

WILL IT COME BACK AGAIN?

Experiencing an episode of depression, at any time in life, increases the likelihood of experiencing further episodes. Research suggests that the *minimum* risk of experiencing a non–childbirth-related episode of illness is 25 per cent (Wisner et al., 2001) and the risk of having another postpartum episode may be as high as 40 per cent, with approximately 24 per cent of all recurrences occurring within the first two weeks postpartum (Wisner et al., 2004).

Are There Effective Treatments for Depression?

Health professionals can effectively treat depression and most women fully recover. Depending on the nature of the illness, treatments can include medication, psychological therapies, counselling and support groups. The different types of treatment available are discussed in detail in Chapter 5.

For a discussion of who to refer to and how to obtain a formal diagnosis of PPD, please see Chapter 6.

RELUCTANCE TO DISCLOSE SYMPTOMS

Women may not be willing to admit to experiencing depressive symptoms for a myriad of reasons, which are discussed in Chapter 3. They may hesitate to talk about how they are feeling because they don't recognize that their symptoms are due to a major mental illness, or because they think they are bad mothers because they are not coping. Or they may feel embarrassed, guilty or resentful, worry about being labelled or stigmatized as mentally ill, or worry that others might minimize or dismiss their fears and concerns. Some cultures do not perceive depression following childbirth as a medical problem that requires intervention. As a result, some women would not seek treatment, or their immediate family would deal with the problem (Oates et al., 2004).

A service provider working with new mothers needs to be aware of the different ways in which depressive symptoms may be presented.

Individuals differ in the *types* of symptoms they experience, the *degree* to which they are affected, and the *manner* and *degree* to which they may disclose symptoms.

Depressive episodes range in severity: some individuals have mild cases through to extremely severe episodes. Irrespective of meeting formal criteria for depression, any woman requires help if she has symptoms that cause her distress, cause problems in her daily living or could become worse.

Different Clinical Presentations of Depressive Symptoms

DEPRESSED MOOD

Women often do not admit to being depressed. They may use other words to convey being depressed, such as despondent, low, sad, irritable, restless, numb or empty. The woman may be tearful or cry more than usual, or say that she is past the stage of crying because she is so empty. Often women express strong feelings of inadequacy, particularly regarding their abilities as a mother, and talk about their inability to cope or fear of being labelled as "a bad mother." They may compare themselves with other new moms or female relatives, which increases their feelings of inadequacy.

In some cases, a woman will not disclose that she has psychological problems but will instead focus on physical symptoms. The mother may complain to her doctor or public health nurse of stomach ache, headache or backache. Some women simply cannot disclose their psychological state, and find that focusing on physical symptoms is a more comfortable means of conveying their distress. Other women will focus on the health of the baby, making repeated visits to the doctor's or nurse's office with physical concerns, even if the doctor or nurse has said that the baby is fine.

Depression with anxiety

It is very common for women experiencing PPD to also exhibit anxiety. Within the context of a PPD, the mother may experience anxiety about the baby's health or her own ability as a mother or concern over how she will cope with childcare responsibilities.

While anxiety is a common feature of depression, some individuals exhibit *only* anxiety. That is, they experience anxious feelings but *do not* have depressed mood or loss of interest or pleasure. (Please see discussion of postpartum anxiety on page 11.)

ANHEDONIA

Women with PPD may lose interest or no longer enjoy activities that used to give them pleasure, such as being with the baby, watching a favourite television program, reading or spending time with a partner, family or friends.

WEIGHT CHANGES AND APPETITE

Health professionals usually define the symptom of weight change as a significant weight gain or loss (in the absence of actively dieting). However, this can be hard to assess in new moms whose weight will change after having a baby. Service providers may prefer to inquire about women's *desire* for and *enjoyment* of food; for example, do they still want food (even if they don't have time to prepare something), do they enjoy it and still like their favourite items?

SLEEP DISTURBANCE

Sleep disturbance is a common symptom of depression. However, this is extremely difficult to gauge in new moms. Service providers may prefer to ask about a mom's ability to sleep or get rest when she has the opportunity—for example, can she sleep when the baby falls asleep; or if someone else is watching the baby, can she sleep, nap or rest? Does she have difficulty falling asleep? Does she wake in the middle of the night and can she fall back to sleep? Does she have difficulty waking up in the morning and does she feel refreshed after sleep?

FATIGUE

It is hard to estimate the real extent of tiredness in new moms. The fatigue associated with depression is a *prevailing* sense of exhaustion *irrespective* of the amount of sleep or rest obtained.

PSYCHOMOTOR RETARDATION OR AGITATION

Psychomotor retardation refers to physical feelings of being slowed down, moving slowly or experiencing sluggishness. Psychomotor agitation refers to feelings of being restless, jumpy and on edge. As well as the mother feeling like this, other people will likely have noticed the movements too, and may have commented on them.

EXCESSIVE FEELINGS OF GUILT OR WORTHLESSNESS

Some individuals have excessive and inappropriate feelings of guilt or worthlessness. This does not just relate to being ill, but is much more severe. They may negatively interpret everyday activities as confirming their low sense of worth; for example, "The other mothers don't talk to me because I don't deserve to have friends because I'm such a bad person." These women may feel guilt to delusional proportions; for example, some women may feel that they are responsible for world poverty or something bad happening to someone else.

DIMINISHED CONCENTRATION, INABILITY TO "THINK STRAIGHT"

Clinicians variously describe lack of concentration as slowed thinking, inability to concentrate on the task at hand, being unable to finish a job or having trouble making simple decisions. Some women complain that they "can't think straight" when confronted by the simplest of tasks.

RECURRENT THOUGHTS OF DEATH OR SUICIDE

Thoughts of death or suicide are a common feature of depressive illness. In many cases, these thoughts express not simply a fear of dying but a preoccupation with death. Women may not explicitly use words such as suicide, death or killing. But they may say things like "The baby and I would be better off dead," or "The world is such an awful place to bring a baby into that we would be better off out of it." Some women feel that they can no longer go on, but cannot bear the thought of leaving the baby behind so would take the baby with them.

Some women have thoughts about hurting the baby that make them feel deeply frightened or ashamed—even though the vast majority would never act on these thoughts. For instance, they might imagine how easy it would be to smother or drown the baby, or throw him or her out of the window. In other cases, women feel it would be a blessing if they went to sleep and didn't wake up, but would not actively do anything to hurt themselves. Some women are obsessed with such thoughts, but most would never act on them. (See Chapter 6.)

Although highly publicized, acts of **infanticide** and suicide are rare in postnatal illness. Infanticide is estimated to occur in one to three in 50,000 births (Brockington & Cox-Roper, 1988; Jason et al., 1983). Health professionals estimate that 62 per cent of mothers who commit infanticide also go on to commit suicide (Gibson, 1982).

Suicide is a risk factor in depressive illness that must be considered. Chapter 6 further discusses assessing risk of suicide.

Other Types of Postpartum Mood Disturbance

In this section we will describe other mood disorders that can occur following childbirth.

Postpartum **affective disorders** generally involve three categories: the blues (baby blues, maternity blues), PPD, and **puerperal**, or postpartum, psychosis, each having different symptoms and severity and requiring different management (see Table 1–1). This section also discusses anxiety following childbirth.

TABLE 1–1

Common Postpartum Mood Disturbances: Summary of Onset, Duration & Treatment

Condition	Prevalence	Onset Often During	Duration	Treatment
Blues	30–75%	Day 3 or 4	Hours to days	No treatment needed other than reassurance
Postpartum Depression	10–15%	Within weeks to 12 months	Weeks to months	Treatment generally required
Puerperal Psychosis	0.1–0.2 %	Within 2 weeks, usually first week	Weeks to months	Hospitalization usually required

Table adapted with permission from Nonacs & Cohen, 1998.

POSTPARTUM, OR "BABY," BLUES

Postpartum blues are the most common perinatal mood disturbance, affecting an estimated 30 to 75 per cent of women. The blues tend to appear in the first few hours to days after birth, usually peaking on day three or four. The symptoms only last a few days and generally cease within a week. Typically, the blues appear in a woman who is happy but experiences increased "emotional" responses to stimuli. She may change rapidly from being happy to tearful, and have inexplicable spells of irritability, weepiness, anxiety and sleep and appetite disturbances. Researchers have suggested that some of these effects may result from the rapid hormonal changes occurring.

The blues are mild, generally requiring no treatment other than support and reassurance. By definition, blues do not last longer than two weeks. And while most women remain well thereafter, up to 20 per cent of women with the blues develop major depression within the first year of having a baby. In some cases, women's symptoms worsen and become depression, while others can recover from the blues and then subsequently experience depression.

POSTPARTUM PINKS

While "the blues" refers to mood lability (or changes in mood from happy to sad), some women experience mild elation, or "the pinks," following childbirth; again, this elation lasts for a few hours to days until a more normal level of happiness returns (Glover et al., 1994). Similar to the baby blues, the pinks do not require treatment, and others may not notice the pinks if they view mild elation as a "normal" reaction to childbirth.

In some situations, symptoms of the blues or pinks require clinical attention. One of the core features of both the blues and pinks is that the mood changes are mild and transient. Extremes of either the blues or pinks are definitely a cause for concern— prolonged mood changes (longer than a few days) or big mood swings from high to low are indications of a more serious mood disorder developing and will require follow-up (see Chapter 6).

POSTPARTUM ANXIETY

As for depression, anxiety occurring around pregnancy or following the birth of a child is *clinically* no different from anxiety that occurs at any other time. However, research data on postpartum anxiety is limited compared with data on other postpartum disorders. Studies indicate that between four and 15 per cent of women experience anxiety following childbirth (Wenzel et al., 2003; Matthey et al., 2003; Heron et al., 2004).

Some women experience anxiety only during pregnancy, some only following childbirth, and others throughout pregnancy and the postpartum period. In a recent large study of 8,323 pregnant British women, Heron et al. (2004) found that 7.3 per cent of women reported high levels of anxiety during pregnancy, as measured by a self-report questionnaire. Of those women who had high levels of anxiety during pregnancy, 1.4 per cent also scored high levels of anxiety when measured at eight weeks postpartum. Of the women who did not report high levels of anxiety during pregnancy, 2.4 per cent reported high levels of anxiety postpartum.

Many mothers feel anxious, overwhelmed and scared following the birth of their baby. This is understandable given the changes involved in becoming a new parent. However, for some women the level of anxiety is so severe that it interferes with their daily lives, and represents a change in normal character and functioning.

DIAGNOSIS

The formal classification of anxiety disorders in the *DSM-IV* covers a range of disorders that may be specific in nature; that is, a specific phobia (such as fear of heights or spiders), panic disorder or obsessive-compulsive disorder. For some people, no one source or situation causes the anxiety, so clinicians consider their condition to be generalized anxiety.

For some women with postpartum anxiety, the fear or anxiety is general, but for others the symptoms may relate to something more specific (i.e., bathing the baby, taking the baby out in the car, coping with grocery shopping) or the symptoms may focus solely on the child (i.e., is the baby feeding properly and breathing properly, is the woman competent as a mother and able to look after the baby?). The mother's anxiety typically exhibits itself as constant and/or excessive worry, fear or apprehension. She may appear edgy, tense and perpetually keyed up. In some cases, women will avoid certain situations because the fear is so overwhelming.

People with anxiety often describe physical symptoms or panic attacks that accompany the anxiety feelings, including:

• sweating
• palpitations
• nausea
• faintness
• an overwhelming urge to run away.

Women with anxiety problems do not experience the persistently low mood and anhedonia (loss of pleasure) that typifies depression, although as previously stated, mothers with PPD may also feel anxious.

PUERPERAL, OR POSTPARTUM, PSYCHOSIS

In contrast to the blues and PPD, postpartum (or puerperal) psychosis is the most severe and rare form of postpartum mood disorder, with rates of one to two episodes per 1,000 deliveries. The onset of symptoms is rapid, in many cases within 48 to 72 hours after birth, and most cases develop within the first two weeks postpartum. Studies (e.g., Jones & Craddock, 2001) suggest that postpartum psychosis has a genetic or biological cause and is more common in women diagnosed with bipolar disorder or with a family history of mood disorders.

The most common symptoms are extreme depressed or elated mood (mania), similar to that seen in bipolar disorder (or manic depression). Women with puerperal psychosis often fluctuate rapidly between mania and depression, or may experience a "high" (mania) followed by a depression. Women often exhibit bizarre or disorganized behaviour, and are often confused or perplexed.

Most women with postpartum psychosis experience psychotic symptoms. Clinicians define **delusions** as false fixed beliefs that have no rational basis in reality and that the individual's culture deems unacceptable. Common types of delusions involve persecution, love and guilt, for example. Clinicians define **hallucinations** as *perceptual distortions* that have no external stimulus. The most common hallucinations are auditory (hearing noises or voices that nobody else hears) or visual (seeing things that are not present and that other people cannot see) (Dubovsky & Buzan, 1999). Examples of psychotic symptoms include the mother believing that she or her baby has special powers or superior intelligence (e.g., the mother believes that she will write a best-selling book or that she is a famous artist, the mother thinks that she and her baby could be on television because they are so talented). Some women may hear voices telling them to do things or saying things to them (which may be positive or negative).

As previously stated, cases of infanticide and suicide are rare but are a serious risk in women with postpartum psychosis. The symptoms of postpartum psychosis fluctuate rapidly, and a woman who was lucid and calm upon first interview can be suicidal and psychotic within a matter of hours.

The nature of the psychosis is very unpredictable and even an experienced **psychiatrist** can have difficulty detecting it (see Spinelli, 2004). Any woman exhibiting extreme mood changes (high to low) or psychotic symptoms requires an immediate emergency psychiatric referral (see Chapter 6).

Summary

PPD is a depressive episode that occurs in the first year postpartum.

Clinically, PPD is no different from depressions occurring at other times, except the symptoms may be related to the birth or baby.

PPD is the most common postpartum mood disorder. It affects approximately 13 per cent of new mothers.

A physician or licensed psychologist makes diagnoses according to *DSM-IV* criteria.

Symptoms of PPD are, predominantly, feelings of sadness and inability to feel pleasure, in addition to sleep disturbance, fatigue, weight change, physical agitation or retardation, excessive feelings of worthlessness or guilt, decreased ability to concentrate and recurrent thoughts of death or suicide.

After having PPD, a woman is at risk of experiencing further depressive episodes related to childbirth, and is also at risk of depression at other times.

Postpartum blues are extremely common in the postpartum period but only last for a few days, and the mood symptoms are mild and transient. PPD is persistent and more severe, lasting a minimum of two weeks and impairing daily functioning.

Women who experience severe elation and depression, or exhibit any psychotic features (postpartum psychosis), require immediate medical and/or psychiatric referral and probably hospital admission.

2

Risk Factors

What causes postpartum depression?

What does it mean if a woman is "at risk" of developing postpartum depression?

What risk factors have researchers associated with postpartum depression?

As previously stated, the postpartum period is a time of increased risk for the development of severe mood disorders in women. While clinicians do not know the **etiology** (or cause) of depression, hypotheses include biological, social and personality models of illness. Because of the massive hormonal fluctuations following childbirth, hormonal models have been suggested as the cause, or triggering mechanism, of the depressive illness. However, current research evidence suggests that one single cause is unlikely. Research also suggests that the triggers of depression, or risk factors, differ between individuals. Genetic and biological studies of mood disorders indicate that they are complex diseases, and even if an individual has a genetic vulnerability or predisposition to developing depression, experiential and environmental factors must interact to cause the illness (Dubovsky & Buzan, 1999). Therefore, the **biopsychosocial model** of illness is the most likely explanation—where biological, social and psychological factors are all involved.

Risk Factors for PPD

Over the last decade or so, many research studies have attempted to identify women who may be at increased risk of developing PPD. Identifying risk factors enables health care professionals working with pregnant women or mothers with new babies to be aware of women who may be more vulnerable to illness. While we still don't know much about which factors may protect against developing PPD, future research may help to identify protective factors.

Nonetheless, it is important to stress that PPD can also occur in women with no known risk factors. Similarly, not all women with risk factors will develop PPD.

Evidence-Based Risk Factors for PPD

The studies presented in this chapter contain results from two large meta-analyses on more than 14,000 subjects (O'Hara & Swain, 1996; Beck, 2001), and results from more recent studies of an additional 10,000 subjects.

The data from these studies show that women with one or more of the risk factors have a *statistically increased* chance of developing PPD compared with women with none of these factors. The strength of the relationships (strong, moderate and weak) derives from a statistical procedure called an effect size. See Figure 2–1.

When interpreting the results of research studies, experts need to consider how the study was designed and conducted. All of the studies discussed in this chapter are **prospective studies**: they include data that researchers collected from a number of women during their pregnancy—or "prospectively"—before the researchers knew who would become depressed. This is the most powerful means of collecting data.

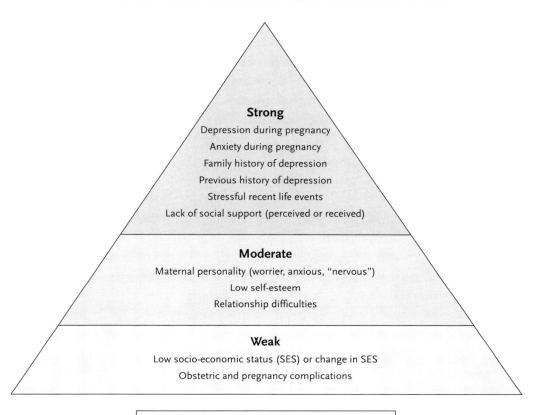

FIGURE 2–1

Evidence-Based Antenatal Risk Factors for PPD

Strong
Depression during pregnancy
Anxiety during pregnancy
Family history of depression
Previous history of depression
Stressful recent life events
Lack of social support (perceived or received)

Moderate
Maternal personality (worrier, anxious, "nervous")
Low self-esteem
Relationship difficulties

Weak
Low socio-economic status (SES) or change in SES
Obstetric and pregnancy complications

No Effect
Ethnicity
Maternal age (except teens)
Sex of child*
Level of education
Number of children

* The sex of the child is not a risk factor within Western societies, but has been found to be an issue in some Asian studies. Studies conducted within Western societies show no association between the sex of the child and depression. Recent studies from Hong Kong (Lee et al., 2000) and India (Patel et al., 2002) have proposed that spousal disappointment with the baby's sex, particularly if the baby is a girl, is significantly associated with developing PPD. Therefore, the parents' reaction to the sex of the baby may be a potential risk factor within certain cultural groups. (See also discussion in Chapter 8.)

Factors Not Associated with Developing PPD

Current research finds the same level of risk applies to individuals across ethnic and racial groups, and all levels of education. Parity, or already having had children, is not protective against depression, but neither does it appear to increase risk. While maternal age is not a risk factor in adult women, the rate of PPD is much higher in teenage mothers (ages 14 to 18 years) than it is in adult mothers: the rate in teenage mothers is 26 per cent (Troutman & Cutrona, 1990) compared with 13 per cent in adult mothers (see Chapter 8).

Strong Predictors of PPD

DEPRESSION OR ANXIETY DURING PREGNANCY

Experiencing a low mood or anxiety during pregnancy is the strongest predictor of PPD. Evaluating results from 25 studies on approximately 12,000 subjects, O'Hara & Swain (1996) and Beck (2001) found that pregnant women who reported depression or anxiety, through questionnaires or clinical interviews, were at high risk of depression following childbirth.

The women who experienced depression or anxiety did not simply have continued symptoms throughout pregnancy and following childbirth; many experienced an episode during pregnancy, recovered and were well for a period of time, and then experienced a subsequent depression following childbirth.

PERSONAL AND FAMILY HISTORY OF MENTAL ILLNESS

Women who have previously had a depressive illness at any time in their lives are at increased risk of developing depression in the postpartum period. In fact, research studies consistently rate a past episode of depression as one of the strongest risk factors for developing PPD. In some cases, the previous history may not be documented, as women may not have sought or received treatment for the depression.

Based on research with women who are known to have experienced an episode of PPD, the risk of experiencing depressive episodes unrelated to childbirth is at least 25 per cent (Wisner et al., 2001) and up to 40 per cent for experiencing further PPD (Wisner et al., 2004).

Current evidence suggests that a family history of psychiatric illness confers an added risk of PPD (Johnstone et al., 2001). Studies examining the effect of a family history of depression in women with PPD have found a higher rate of mental illness within close relatives (Steiner & Tam, 1999; Steiner, 2002; O'Hara et al., 1984). Studies have repeatedly shown that mood disorders tend to run in families. First-degree relatives (parents, children or siblings) of individuals with depression have a 5.5 per cent to 28.4 per cent risk of depression themselves. However, researchers do not know whether this is due to genetic transmission or to a shared family environment.

One difficulty in evaluating the influence of a family history of mental illness on PPD is that the woman concerned must know her family history (which she may not) and be willing to disclose it. Due to the high prevalence of depressive illness in the general population, many women will have at least one relative who has a history of depression. Researchers think that having several first-degree (close) relatives with this illness may increase the likelihood of developing PPD.

STRESSFUL LIFE EVENTS

Studies have clearly established that depression often occurs following adverse or stressful life events, such as the death of a loved one, divorce, relationship breakups, a job change or moving house, immigrating or becoming a **refugee**. These events are recognized **stressors** that can precipitate depressive symptoms even in people with no previous history of mood disorders.

Study design is crucial in clarifying the relationship between life events and PPD. Retrospective data gathering, or collecting information *after* the baby's birth, can lead to overreporting of life events, with subjects (perhaps subconsciously) trying to link a past stressful experience to their current depression. Collecting the data during the woman's pregnancy avoids this bias. Research shows that women who experience a stressful life event during pregnancy are more likely to develop PPD.

LACK OF SOCIAL SUPPORT

Receiving social support during stressful times is highly protective against depression. Studies show a correlation between depressive illness and social support both during pregnancy and in the immediate postpartum period (Beck, 1996; Menaghann, 1990; Seguin et al., 1999). The evidence clearly suggests that women who feel that they lack social support are at increased risk of developing PPD.

Social support is a multidimensional concept. Sources of support can be a spouse or partner, relatives or friends. There are also different types of social support, including *informational* support (provision of sound advice and guidance), *instrumental* support (practical assistance with everyday baby-caring and household tasks) and *emotional* support (expressions of love, care and sympathy).

Studies have consistently shown that a *perceived* lack of social support during pregnancy is a strong risk factor for PPD (Seguin et al., 1999; Forman et al., 2000). Often if a woman is depressed, a discrepancy may exist between her *perceived* support (her own view or perception of the support she gets) and the support that she actually *receives* (which can be objectively assessed).

The support traditionally offered to pregnant women and new moms varies widely in different cultures and societies. Although human pregnancy and childbirth are physiologically the same worldwide, the concepts and traditions surrounding them vary widely in different populations.

In some societies, and in some communities in Canada, a woman traditionally returns to the parental home for a few weeks after delivery, likely assuring her of adequate assistance with the new infant. Likewise, a family member may stay with the newborn and parent(s) in their own home for a few weeks to offer support. By contrast, recent **immigrants** who have few relatives nearby may feel very isolated in their new country, with less social support than they would get back home (Oates et al., 2004). Separated from a family that would normally provide assistance, these women may be especially vulnerable to PPD (see also Chapter 8).

Moderate Risk Factors

PSYCHOLOGICAL RISK FACTORS

Maternal personality characteristics including **neuroticism**, low self-esteem and negative **cognitive** (or thinking) styles are considered moderate risk factors for PPD.

While psychiatrists no longer professionally use the term "neurotic," it still commonly appears in questionnaires. Clinicians generally regard neurotic disorders as a dysfunctional way of dealing with anxiety, and although the person can still think rationally and function socially, such disorders cause distress. Studies have found that women identified through questionnaires as "nervous," as "shy–self-conscious" or as "worriers" have significantly elevated risks of developing PPD (Johnstone et al., 2001).

Similarly, studies find that women with negative cognitive (thinking) styles have elevated risks of developing PPD. Negative cognitive styles include being prone to pessimism, anger or rumination (endless mulling over failings or self-criticism). The findings suggest that psychological symptoms seen after childbirth may have origins preceding the woman's pregnancy.

Experiencing marital or relationship discord during pregnancy can put women at increased risk of PPD. Studies have shown that a poor relationship or conflicts with the baby's father (or current partner) exacerbate PPD or increase the risk of developing this illness. This is closely linked with the findings on social support, where lacking emotional, practical and informational support, particularly from a partner, can lead to depression. A close, supportive relationship with the baby's father (or with a current partner) both during pregnancy and after childbirth can help to mitigate the stress of new parenthood. (For a full discussion of issues relating to relationships, please see Chapter 7.)

Weak Risk Factors

OBSTETRIC FACTORS

Results from meta-analyses show that pregnancy and delivery complications play a small but significant role in the development of PPD. These obstetric factors can include pregnancy-related complications, such as **pre-eclampsia**, hyperemesis and premature contractions, as well as delivery-related complications, such as Caesarean section, use of forceps, premature delivery and excessive intrapartum bleeding. However, research has not yet clarified whether or not the obstetric complications and manner of birth increase the risk of PPD, or whether prolonged hospitalization and bedrest contribute to the depressed mood.

The evidence about the relationship between PPD and delivery by Caesarean section is contradictory and underlines the need for caution in interpreting the data, particularly given the wide variance in Caesarean section rates in different geographical areas, different hospitals and certainly between countries. Several recent studies have suggested that women who undergo *emergency* Caesarean deliveries are more likely to become depressed than those who have elective Caesarean sections (Boyce & Todd, 1992).

Reports on the link between PPD and unplanned or unwanted pregnancies and breastfeeding also differ. Some studies suggest that not breastfeeding at six weeks postpartum confers some extra risk of PPD, while others dispute this idea. Since attitudes toward and rates of breastfeeding differ within populations, cultures and countries, results understandably diverge. Other confounding variables may include the woman with depression deciding not to breastfeed, perhaps due to fatigue, or because she is taking medications.

Service providers should exercise caution in interpreting studies regarding unwanted or unplanned pregnancies and the onset of depression; the fact that the woman did not plan the pregnancy merely reflects the circumstances in which conception occurred, and is not a measure of the woman's feelings toward the fetus.

SOCIO-ECONOMIC STATUS

The role of socio-economic status in the etiology of mental health disorders has received much attention. Researchers have cited indicators of socio-economic deprivation, such as unemployment, low income and low education, as risk factors in mental health disorders, and in depression in particular (World Health Organization, 2001). The evidence suggests that socio-economic factors play a small but significant role in the development of PPD. Low income, unemployment, financial strain and mother's occupation are possible predictors of PPD (O'Hara & Swain, 1996; Warner et al., 1996).

Clinical Overview

Although no typical model exists for a woman at risk of developing PPD, O'Hara and his colleagues (O'Hara et al., 1996) produced a "clinical composite" that is useful for service providers working with pregnant women and new mothers. According to this clinical composite, a woman at risk of developing PPD may have had previous episodes of psychiatric illness, although she may not have sought help for depressive symptoms. She may have experienced an episode of depression or anxiety during pregnancy, which may have been dismissed as "hormonal" or may not have been recognized as being due to a serious illness. She may be experiencing difficulties through stressful life events and a poor relationship with her partner. And she may think that her partner, family and friends are not as supportive as they could be, or she may not have any family or close friends who can provide support. A woman who has experienced any of the risk factors for PPD is more vulnerable to developing the illness.

Summary

There is no single risk factor for PPD.

While experts have long suspected that hormonal variables play a role in precipitating PPD, current evidence suggests that social and psychological factors play an equal or greater role.

As with depression that occurs at other times in life, various factors can contribute to PPD.

The strongest risk factors for PPD are:
- symptoms of depression or anxiety during pregnancy
- a history of depression, in the woman or her immediate family members
- a lack of social support
- recent stressful life events (e.g., moving house, relationship breakdown, death of a loved one).

If a woman has one or more of the above risk factors, she is statistically more likely to develop an episode of PPD than is a woman without any risk factors.

However, many women with risk factors do not develop PPD, and occasionally, women with no risk factors do develop PPD.

Knowing which women are most "at risk" may help caregivers decide when screening for PPD may be worthwhile. (See also Chapter 3.)

3
Detection and Screening

Why does postpartum depression often remain undetected?

What is screening?

What criteria should be considered when deciding whether or not to develop a screening program?

What tools do clinicians use to detect postpartum depression?

When would be the most effective time to screen for postpartum depression?

Do new mothers benefit from postpartum depression screening?

Should service providers screen women for postpartum depression?

There is mounting interest in methods to detect **postpartum depression (PPD)** due to the negative consequences for both the mother and her family. However, determining the best way to identify mothers who are either at risk for PPD or currently experiencing depressive symptoms is challenging. This chapter reviews the issues that impede the detection of PPD, and the potential role for screening programs in improving its detection. It describes the two main types of screening procedures—targeted and universal—and outlines important issues that inform decisions about screening programs. This includes examining the merits of currently available PPD screening tools and the debates about the optimal time to screen for PPD.

The authors cannot recommend routine, universal screening for PPD at this time, as there is still not enough research to support a link between screening and improved outcomes for mothers. However, we felt that it was important to describe screening procedures and identify the gaps in existing research related to PPD screening, as screening is being conducted in some health care units and agencies across Canada.

Difficulties in Detecting PPD

Despite the long-standing recognition of PPD, the condition remains largely undetected. There are many reasons for this. First, women are often reluctant to seek professional help (Small et al., 1994). Even though mothers interact with various service providers in the postpartum period, mothers are frequently unwilling to disclose emotional problems, particularly depression (Brown & Lumley, 2000). Their reticence to disclose their true feelings may in part be due to the popular myth that equates motherhood with happiness, along with the idealization of the "good mother," which emphasizes feelings of joy while minimizing those of unhappiness. In addition, many women assume the struggles they are experiencing are a normal part of motherhood. These women may attribute their symptoms to causes other than depression, such as fatigue or relationship difficulties (Small et al., 1994; Whitton et al., 1996). Conversely, some women recognize the symptoms as depression but fear that, if they seek help, they will be labelled as mentally ill or as unfit mothers. Furthermore, clinicians have observed that many mothers do not disclose their feelings of depression because they are afraid that child welfare staff will remove their child from the family home.

Even after women have decided to seek professional help, service providers may minimize their symptoms or portray their experiences as normal, leaving mothers feeling embarrassed, disappointed or frustrated (Beck, 1993). Not knowing where to obtain assistance is another important barrier to seeking help (McIntosh, 1993). Family members may also discourage women from seeking help, as in some cultures it is particularly unacceptable to admit to having depressive symptoms to someone outside of the family. Finally, one area identified as a key reason for mothers not seeking mental health care is that help is not available in their language; this is true for French-speaking Canadians living in areas of the country where they are a minority group, as well as for non–English-speaking **immigrant** populations. In addition to linguistic gaps in service, some women feel that service providers will not respect their cultural beliefs and traditions.

Service providers may also contribute to the underdiagnosing of PPD. Many service providers have limited training in assessing or managing PPD. As such, they often do not ask mothers about their mood or recognize the mother's symptoms as indicating depression. Alternatively, they may feel uncertain about how to effectively help and so are reluctant to raise such issues.

SUMMARY OF BARRIERS TO PPD DETECTION

Barriers to mothers recognizing or disclosing PPD:
- believing the popular myth that equates motherhood with happiness
- assuming that their struggles are a normal part of motherhood
- fearing such labels as "mentally ill" or "unfit mother," and believing that they could result in someone taking away their child
- not knowing where and how to obtain help
- family members discouraging them from seeking help.

Barriers to health care providers identifying PPD:
- failing to assess for PPD
- minimizing symptoms of depression
- limited training or expertise in detecting and managing PPD
- not knowing how to effectively help, so reluctant to raise issues
- services not culturally sensitive
- services not available in the person's language, making the expression of emotion difficult.

What Is Screening?

Screening describes a systematic process used to detect diseases or conditions, including PPD. It involves the use of tools or procedures applied to a defined population (e.g., new mothers). The purpose of these tools or procedures is to detect an unrecognized disorder or condition in individuals who do not yet perceive that they are at risk of, or suspect that they are affected by, a condition or its complications (e.g., depression). In screening programs, clinicians ask people a question or offer them a tool, such as a questionnaire, that they can complete on their own. How people respond to the questions in the questionnaire determines whether or not they are likely to benefit from further examination or appropriate treatment.

Screening tools do not diagnose a condition but rather only identify individuals who are at risk of developing the condition or are displaying potential symptoms of the condition. In the case of PPD, for example, service providers could use screening procedures to identify women whom they should refer for further assessment and possible diagnosis of PPD by a mental health specialist.

There are two main types of screening: targeted screening and universal screening. Through "targeted" screening procedures, only individuals identified as being at increased risk for the disease or condition in question undergo screening. Clinicians usually identify these individuals as being at increased risk in one of two ways:
- The individuals themselves, their family members, or their health or social service providers recognize symptoms of the disease or condition.

- A clinician finds that the individual has one or more risk factors for the disease or condition, as identified through the clinical assessment or use of a screening tool that is not disease-specific and is used in general clinical practice. One such screening tool is the Antenatal Psychosocial Health Assessment (ALPHA) form, which Ontario physicians caring for pregnant women may have completed. This form includes a depression item and examines 15 psychosocial risk factors, grouped into four categories: family dynamics, maternal factors, substance use and family violence.

With "universal" screening procedures, all members of the defined population (e.g., new mothers) are screened. Universal screening procedures have the potential to detect every case of a disease/condition but require substantial resources to implement. Due to the significant costs associated with universal screening programs, service providers generally do not undertake them without substantial research evidence that the screening will ultimately improve the health of the population being screened.

Because fewer individuals are examined, targeted screening procedures are usually less costly and therefore more feasible in many settings. However, because not every person in the population undergoes screening, health care providers are more likely to miss cases of the disease or condition with targeted screening than with universal screening procedures. The number of people who will go undetected with targeted screening depends on the condition in question. No one knows how many women with PPD would remain undetected in a targeted PPD screening program.

Screening has the potential to save lives or improve the quality of life through early diagnosis of a serious condition. However, screening is not perfect: in any screening program, whether universal or targeted, there will always be a certain number of *false positive* results (individuals wrongly reported to have the condition) and *false negative* results (individuals wrongly reported as *not* having the condition).

Criteria for a Screening Program

To assist service providers in developing effective universal or targeted screening programs, specific criteria exist related to (1) the disorder or condition; (2) the screening tool; and (3) the health care system (see Table 3–1) (Wilson & Junger, 1968).

CONDITION CRITERIA

Service providers should only use screening procedures to detect conditions that are deemed important health problems. If a condition is extremely rare, the cost and effort of screening may be prohibitive. As a result, service providers need to know the prevalence of the condition in a population before embarking on any large-scale screening program. They should also have reason to expect that early detection and management of the condition they are assessing will benefit the individuals in question. Finally, effective treatment for individuals with the condition should be available.

PPD meets some of these criteria. It affects approximately 13 per cent of all new mothers, making it an important public health issue, and research suggests that effective treatment does exist (see Chapter 5). However, treatment options are not readily available to some mothers, especially those in rural and remote settings. Nonetheless, early detection may assist mothers to access available treatment and potentially diminish the possibility of long-term adverse effects.

SCREENING TOOL CRITERIA

Screening tools should accurately identify individuals with the condition or those who are at risk of developing it. They should be safe, convenient and acceptable to women, as well as cost-effective, easy to interpret and readily incorporated into practice. The tools should also be validated in other languages besides English.

Several screening tools can be used to identify women with PPD. (See page 30.) These tools have been assessed for accuracy against diagnostic clinical interviews and can be easily integrated into practice with proper planning. Research also suggests that women are receptive to PPD screening procedures. However, most screening tools have been assessed for accuracy with primarily Caucasian mothers or native-born women (e.g., the tool was tested among Chinese women in China or Hong Kong). Limited work has been conducted to evaluate the accuracy of these screening tools in immigrant women or multicultural populations. Additional research is also needed to determine which mode of administration (e.g., face-to-face, telephone, self-administered) is most accurate and preferred among the various cultures.

HEALTH CARE SYSTEM CRITERIA

Several health care system criteria should be included in a screening program. In essence, these criteria are designed to ensure that individuals who screen positive for the disease or condition in question will receive appropriate and effective care as a result. For example, an effective treatment should exist for individuals identified through early detection, with evidence that early treatment leads to better outcomes than late treatment. The agency or health unit should establish agreed-upon evidence-based policies for referral and preventive/treatment options that are accessible and acceptable before a screening program is initiated.

Furthermore, responsibilities in the screening program should be clear (i.e., who does what and when). Those administering the screening program also need to outline how the findings will become part of a participant's medical record. And issues around confidentiality need to be addressed. The costs of the screening program (including testing, diagnosis and treatment) should be economically balanced in relation to the cost of health care as a whole. Once the program is established, ongoing monitoring and evaluation should be incorporated. For additional general information about these health care system criteria, readers can refer to Muir-Gray (2001), Cadman et al. (1984) and Sackett (1987).

These health care system criteria are less developed than the other criteria for PPD. In many communities, few effective options are available for treating or preventing PPD. Service providers should not begin screening for PPD until there are services where women suspected to have PPD can be referred. The few PPD screening programs that do exist have not yet been evaluated to the extent that their findings can inform others about the costs and benefits of screening. *As such, limited research exists to assist providers in integrating these health care system criteria into an efficient and effective screening program.* This is a serious limitation, since screening experts suggest that public health interventions such as screening should undergo the same rigorous evaluations as clinical interventions. They also argue that evidence is needed to support introducing screening to healthy populations, since this kind of intervention can be burdensome to people without any identifiable problem. As such, additional research is greatly needed to guide the development of PPD screening programs.

TABLE 3–1

Screening Program Criteria and Relationship to PPD

Condition Issues	Does PPD Meet This Criterion?
• The condition should be an important health problem.	Yes
• The progression of the condition should be understood.	Yes
• Effective treatment for individuals with the condition should be available.	While effective treatment does exist, resources are not widely available.
Screening Tool Issues	
• Screening tools should have good sensitivity, specificity and predictive value.	Tools have primarily been evaluated with Caucasian women; researchers need more information about multicultural populations and immigrant women.

• The screening procedure should be safe, convenient and acceptable to the target population.	Yes
• Screening tools should be cost-effective, easy to interpret and readily incorporated into practice.	Yes
• Screening tools should be accessible to the target population.	Not all tools have been translated and validated.
Health Care System Issues	
• Effective treatment should exist for patients identified through early detection, with evidence that early treatment leads to better outcomes than late treatment. • Policies should stipulate what action to take for borderline results in order to avoid overidentifying the condition. • Agreed-upon evidence-based policies for accessible and acceptable referral, prevention and treatment options should be established. • Facilities for screening, diagnosis and treatment should be available, as the lack of follow-up negates the benefit of screening. • Responsibilities in the screening program should be clear (i.e., who does what and when). • Guidelines should specify how the findings will become part of a participant's medical record. • The costs of the screening program (including testing, diagnosis and treatment) should be economically balanced in relation to the cost of health care as a whole. • Compliance with an effective care pathway should be ensured; otherwise, screening offers no benefit (i.e., if someone scores positive, then that person should receive the care suggested by the screening policies). • The screening program should incorporate continuous monitoring and evaluation. • Screening programs should be modified based on current research.	Systematic data is not yet available; data varies from region to region.

In summary, PPD partially meets the condition and screening tool criteria required to establish a screening program. However, PPD has not met health care system criteria, as no economic evaluation of a PPD screening program (including testing, diagnosis and treatment) has taken place. However, the degree to which PPD has met referral policy and treatment availability criteria will vary from setting to setting: some communities may have a well-developed referral network and effective and accessible treatment options in place, while others may be just beginning to identify the needs of postpartum women or have limited resources to address these needs. Service providers need to carefully consider the degree to which these health care system criteria are met in each area before deciding to implement a screening program. Essentially, women should not undergo screening for PPD until it is certain that each woman who screens positive will have timely access to appropriate and effective treatment and prevention resources. In rural or remote areas, these resources may be very limited.

Screening Tools Used to Detect PPD

The most common and clinically useful way to screen for depressive symptoms among new mothers is to administer a self-report questionnaire. Several self-report questionnaires exist for women to rate the frequency or severity of their own depressive symptoms. Screening tools are not intended to diagnose clinical depression. The aim of screening tools is to identify possible symptoms of depression and determine whether or not a service provider needs to do further evaluation—they do not substitute for a diagnosis, which requires a full clinical evaluation. For more details about how to obtain a diagnosis of PPD, please refer to Chapter 6.

THE EDINBURGH POSTNATAL DEPRESSION SCALE (EPDS)

By far the most widely used self-report questionnaire for PPD is the **Edinburgh Postnatal Depression Scale (EDPS)** (Cox et al., 1987). The EPDS is a 10-item questionnaire that is distributed free-of-charge and has been effectively used internationally to assess mothers for depressive symptoms (see Appendix A, page 151). A health care provider typically administers the questionnaire postnatally at varying time periods. Each item is scored on a four-point scale from 0 to 3, with a total score ranging from 0 to 30. The items include questions referring to maternal feelings during the past seven days, asking about depressed mood, **anhedonia** (inability to feel pleasure), guilt, anxiety and self-harming thoughts.

Research suggests that a score of 13 or higher on the EPDS signifies symptoms of major depression. A woman scoring 10 or higher is recommended for community-based screening (i.e., screening conducted among a general population of mothers who may or may not have depressive symptoms) to avoid missing any women with depression or those at risk to develop PPD (Cox et al., 1987). In general, any mother who scores 10 or higher on the EPDS should be referred to a qualified service provider for further assessment (see Appendix B, page 153).

One advantage of the EPDS is that, unlike other depression rating scales, it does not ask about somatic symptoms such as insomnia and appetite changes, which affect almost all new mothers during the postpartum period. Only one item on the EPDS addresses a somatic symptom: "I have been so unhappy that I have had difficulty in sleeping." However, the lack of questions about somatic symptoms on the EPDS may also be a disadvantage, as a subgroup of women with PPD appears to present primarily with physical or somatic complaints rather than psychological symptoms (Ross et al., 2003).

Another advantage of the EPDS is that it is available in more than 23 languages, and researchers from various disciplines have evaluated its screening accuracy. Although researchers have suggested slightly different EPDS cut-off scores for several translated versions, discrepancies in cut-off scores are a problem with most translated tools, not just the EPDS. A recent review of the EPDS outlines these culturally specific cut-off scores (Eberhard-Gran et al., 2002). Chapter 8 addresses how to use the EPDS and other screening tools in women from diverse cultures. However, most research validating the EPDS among diverse cultures has not involved women who have left their native country and have immigrated to a new country. Also, no one has tested the EPDS in a large multicultural population.

Despite these limitations, the EPDS is an internationally recognized tool that has been widely used by researchers and health care providers to assess for depressive symptoms among new mothers. Researchers and health care providers have found the EPDS to be (1) convenient to administer (requires little time or special training and can even be done via telephone), (2) inoffensive to women (high acceptability in diverse cultures) and (3) readily incorporated into everyday clinical practice.

POSTPARTUM DEPRESSION SCREENING SCALE (PDSS)

The **Postpartum Depression Screening Scale (PDSS)** is a newer 35-item depression rating scale (Beck & Gable, 2000). It consists of seven dimensions, each containing five items, and requires a fee for use. The tool is generally administered by service providers early in the postpartum period (around six weeks after delivery). The items examined in the PDSS include sleeping and eating disturbances, anxiety and insecurity, emotional swings, **cognitive** impairment, loss of self, guilt and shame and contemplating harming oneself. Each of the 35 items describes how a woman may feel after the birth of her baby. Respondents indicate the extent to which they agree or disagree with each statement using a five-point scale to rate their feelings during the past two weeks.

A PDSS cut-off score of 80 indicates major depressive symptoms and a cut-off score of 60 indicates probable depressive symptoms. To date, however, very few published studies have compared the PDSS and EPDS to determine which scale is more accurate in detecting PPD (Beck & Gable, 2001a; Beck & Gable, 2001b). The PDSS is a newly developed instrument, so it is only now being translated into different languages and its acceptability in diverse cultures remains unknown. Only a few researchers, and primarily the developer, have thus far evaluated the tool's screening accuracy and additional independent research is greatly needed.

OTHER TOOLS

In addition to the EPDS, the PDSS and other self-report screening tools, a number of standardized interviews and special clinician-rated scales are available to detect depression (although not specifically PPD). Trained clinicians or researchers who have a thorough knowledge of diagnostic systems such as the *DSM-IV* typically use these for research purposes. These instruments (e.g., Hamilton Depression Rating Scale for Depression or Montgomery-Asberg Depression Rating Scale) are not recommended for general clinical practice.

A Few Points to Consider When Using Screening Tools

Some researchers and clinicians (Elliott & Leverton, 2000) have identified common misperceptions about how to use and interpret PPD screening tools. Below are a few mistakes to avoid:

- *"A score below a cut-off confirms that the mother has no mental health disorder."* Using the EPDS as an example, it is unlikely that a mother scoring below 10 has clinically significant levels of depression. However, it is possible, particularly when the tool is administered to multicultural populations. Furthermore, service providers need to recognize that a low score on the EPDS does not rule out symptoms of other mental health conditions or problems of concern (e.g., anxiety disorders or **psychosis**).
- *"Women can pass or fail a screening test."* Screening tools such as the EPDS yield a range of scores on a continuum of maternal distress. The choice of a cut-off score is to some extent arbitrary, and depends on the purpose of the screening process. If the person administering the tool is doing so to confirm depressive symptoms in order to initiate treatment, then an EPDS score of more than 13 may be appropriate. However, if the purpose of the screening process is to identify mothers with potential PPD in order to provide additional assessment, or if it is being used in community-based screening to identify mothers with identified risk factors for PPD, then an EPDS score of more than nine may be appropriate. In other words, there is no one screening tool score below which women have "failed" the test.

- *"The screening tool makes the decision to treat, so a score above the cut-off point means a referral to a service provider."* An EPDS score is only one factor to consider when deciding on whether or not to initiate treatment and preventive strategies. Clinical judgment also plays a critical role. Finally, it is important that the decision be a collaborative one between the mother and her service provider.

When to Screen for PPD

SCREENING IN THE ANTENATAL PERIOD

In the past few decades, many screening tools have been tested to determine whether or not they can be used during pregnancy to predict which women will develop PPD. An excellent review of 16 antenatal screening studies conducted in several countries (including the United Kingdom, Portugal, Australia, Sweden and Denmark) found that antenatal testing missed many women who subsequently developed PPD, and many women identified as "at risk" during pregnancy did not become depressed in the postpartum period (Austin & Lumley, 2003). *Although antenatal screening may raise awareness about PPD for the woman and her health care providers, the research evidence clearly shows that antenatal screening cannot reliably identify women at risk for developing future PPD. It is therefore not recommended as part of routine prenatal care.*

However, approximately 12 per cent of women are depressed during pregnancy (Bennett et al., 2004), and the EPDS *can* detect depressive symptoms in the pregnant mother. Therefore, when the health care system criteria described above are met, a health unit or organization might decide to use the EPDS or another screening tool to identify pregnant women for *current* depression, so that these women receive treatment as soon as possible.

So long as the goal is to detect *current* rather than *future* depression, screening tools can be useful during the antenatal period. When deciding whether or not to implement routine antenatal screening for current depression, service providers must use the same criteria described in this chapter for postpartum screening. However, since even fewer research studies have examined the effectiveness of antenatal screening programs, there is insufficient evidence to determine whether or not screening for depression during pregnancy will actually improve outcomes for mothers (please see below, "Do New Mothers Benefit from PPD Screening?").

SCREENING IN THE POSTPARTUM PERIOD

Traditionally, experts have proposed that screening tools be administered between six and eight weeks postpartum. The rationale for waiting to screen until six weeks postpartum is that the symptoms of the baby blues will have resolved by this time. Screening earlier in the postpartum period might result in a high false positive rate (i.e., wrongly identifying women with PPD when they actually have symptoms of the blues and will likely recover without treatment). In the Canadian health care system, a benefit of screening at approximately six weeks postpartum is that most women will attend a follow-up appointment with their obstetrical health care provider around this time, and therefore may be relatively easy to access.

More recently, some researchers and health care providers have suggested that even despite the high false positive rate, screening during the immediate postpartum period (i.e., the first two weeks postpartum) may be preferred to waiting until six to eight weeks postpartum. Strong research evidence suggests that low maternal mood in the immediate postpartum period (first two weeks postpartum) is highly predictive of the development of PPD (Hannah et al., 1992; Hapgood et al., 1988; Teissedre & Chabrol, 2004; Yamashita et al., 2000; Yoshida et al., 1997). For example, in a population-based sample of 594 Canadian mothers who completed the EPDS at one, four and eight weeks postpartum, the one-week EPDS score accurately identified more than 80 per cent of the mothers with depressive symptoms at four and eight weeks postpartum (Dennis, 2004a). Based on these results, screening in the immediate postpartum period (with appropriate follow-up to confirm that the depressive symptoms identified in the initial screening do meet criteria for the diagnosis of PPD) may be a very useful way to accurately identify mothers who could benefit from PPD treatment.

The obvious benefit of screening during the immediate postpartum period is that women who are already depressed at two weeks postpartum will receive treatment much earlier than if screening did not occur until six weeks postpartum. Early detection and treatment has important benefits for the mother and her family, as described in Chapter 5. The primary disadvantage of screening in the immediate postpartum period is that a significant proportion of the women who screen positive for depression at one to two weeks postpartum may not meet diagnostic criteria for depression, and therefore, women who do not actually require treatment for PPD might consume substantial resources. Where resources permit, however, a two-stage screening process, in which mothers who score positive during the first screening assessment take the screening tool again at a later date, may be the most effective way to implement a screening program. Research has not determined exactly how much later to administer the screening tool again.

There is no research specifying exactly when in the postpartum period to administer these screening tools. However, it is unlikely that there is a *critical* time for screening. Given the lack of research, it seems reasonable that if health care providers are to implement a screening program, they should base the decision as to when to administer the screening tool on (1) their current standards of care and (2) the time when they can reach the most new mothers possible.

Do New Mothers Benefit from PPD Screening?

While universal and targeted screening for PPD may help to identify women with depressive symptoms who need assistance, the benefits of PPD screening have only been partially explored. And significant gaps exist in the literature related to other important outcomes. For example, few studies have evaluated the effect of screening on the number of women who receive appropriate treatment (Schaper et al., 1994).

DOES PPD SCREENING INCREASE THE NUMBER OF MOTHERS WITH DEPRESSIVE SYMPTOMS WHO RECEIVE APPROPRIATE TREATMENT?

The link between PPD screening and the receipt of treatment has not been clearly demonstrated. In the general (non-postpartum) depression literature, a systematic review (Pignone et al., 2002) reported several studies that found screening did not lead to a significant increase in the number of patients treated for depression (Dowrick, 1995; Linn & Yager, 1980; Williams et al., 1999). Another study in this systematic review noted that screening increased the number of antidepressant prescriptions but not the number of referrals for counselling or psychiatric care (Callahan et al., 1994); one study found screening led to only a 10 per cent increase in appropriate treatment (Wells et al., 2000). These results suggest that the link between depression screening and the receipt of appropriate treatment is not strong or consistent. Researchers need to conduct more studies specifically related to depression in postpartum women.

DOES PPD SCREENING INCREASE THE NUMBER OF MOTHERS WHO RECOVER FROM PPD?

Like the receipt of appropriate treatment, the link between PPD screening and an increase in the number of mothers who recover from PPD has not been clearly demonstrated. In the literature about general depression, the effect of screening on recovery from depression is highly variable. In a review examining screening for depression in adults (Pignone et al., 2002), two small trials found that screening produced a significant decrease in the number of patients experiencing major depression at a later time (Johnstone & Goldberg, 1976; Zung & King, 1983). However, two larger trials found screening led to only moderate improvements in depression remission (Wells et al., 2000; Williams et al., 1999), and four other studies found small or no improvements in the number of patients experiencing depressive symptoms at a later time (Callahan et al., 1996; Callahan et al., 1994; Reifler et al., 1996; Whooley et al., 2000). The overall results suggest only a weak link between screening and increased remission rates from depression.

In summary, no research studies to date have investigated the extent to which PPD screening will ultimately improve the mental health of postpartum women. Research on men and women with depression outside of the postpartum period has shown disappointing results so far: screening has not consistently increased either the number of people who receive treatment for depression or the number of patients who go on to recover from their depression.

A number of reasons may explain why screening is not resulting in the hoped-for long-term outcomes. In the case of PPD, the problems are probably not related to the process of screening *per se:* research suggests that incorporating a screening tool such as the EPDS into clinical practice does improve the ability of health care providers to identify women who may have PPD (Evins et al., 2000; Fergerson et al., 2002). However, once health care providers have identified women with possible PPD, the degree to which they can offer the women appropriate treatment is likely highly variable depending on the resources and expertise available. *More research and consistent access to appropriate treatment programs are needed before health professionals can recommend the implementation of a universal or targeted screening program to improve the mental health of mothers.*

Should Service Providers Screen Women for PPD?

Universal screening programs are associated with very significant costs. These costs include not only economic burden, but also the potential harm in identifying a woman who may have PPD and not providing her with access to effective treatment options. In addition, there are costs associated with false positive results (i.e., incorrectly identifying a woman as possibly having PPD), including the potential for labelling and **stigmatization** (Austin & Lumley, 2003; McLennan & Offord, 2002; Pignone et al., 2002).

Based on the lack of evidence that screening will improve the mental health of mothers, and considering the substantial cost associated with implementing a universal screening program, the authors cannot recommend universal screening programs for PPD at this time. With continued research and clinical practice, the quality of care received by women with possible PPD will hopefully improve to the extent that the benefits from a universal screening program will become clear. Until this research is completed, however, the costs of universal screening for PPD outweigh the potential benefits.

In areas where resources are available, however, many service providers are eager to implement some form of screening program to improve their ability to identify women with possible PPD. Some health units and organizations with substantial economic and treatment resources may choose to be leaders in conducting the necessary research to examine the potential benefits of a universal screening program. Others may find a targeted screening approach to be more feasible for them (e.g., administering the EPDS only to those women with a high score on a psychosocial assessment).

Should service providers decide to implement a screening program, whether universal or targeted, they must plan carefully to ensure that the screening tool and health care system criteria described above are met *before* screening begins. Specifically, they will need to:

- evaluate the accuracy of the screening tool if they are using it with a multicultural population or with immigrant mothers
- develop strategies to ensure that the screening program will reach all high-risk mothers (For example, how will they reach mothers who do not attend their six-week postpartum checkup, or decline a postpartum visit by a public health nurse?)
- create evidence-based protocols to connect women who screen positive with appropriate treatment or prevention strategies (see Chapters 4 and 5)
- clearly outline who will be responsible for identifying mothers to be screened (in a targeted screening program, on the basis of specified risk factors or their score on a psychosocial assessment), who will administer the PPD screening tool and who will have access to the results
- develop guidelines to evaluate the screening program for beneficial effects, such as the number of women who received appropriate treatment and those who are no longer depressed at a specific time (e.g., 12 weeks postpartum or X weeks after the initiation of treatment)
- develop strategies to minimize the potentially harmful effects of screening described above, possibly including a public education campaign to decrease the effects of potential labelling and stigma associated with PPD
- examine the cost of a screening program to ensure that it is an appropriate use of limited resources.

In summary, no easy answer exists to the question, "Should service providers screen women for PPD?" The answer will very much depend on the PPD-related resources and expertise in each service provider's area and his or her ability to integrate an evaluation component to demonstrate the benefits of the screening program. A careful weighing of the risks and benefits of screening, including the important screening tool and health care criteria discussed in this chapter, will help service providers to determine whether or not it is appropriate to implement and evaluate a screening program in their area.

Summary

PPD continues to go largely undetected due to both maternal factors (e.g., the "good mother" myth, the fear of being labelled) and health care provider factors (e.g., lack of knowledge of PPD).

Screening describes a systematic process used to detect diseases or conditions, including PPD. It involves the use of tools or procedures applied to a defined population (e.g., new mothers), in order to detect an unrecognized disorder or condition in individuals who do not yet perceive they are at risk of, or suspect that they are affected by, a condition or its complications (e.g., depression). Screening procedures are either "universal," wherein all members of the defined population undergo screening, or "targeted," wherein only individuals identified as being at increased risk for the condition undergo screening.

Specific criteria exist to help health care providers develop effective screening procedures related to (1) the condition itself (e.g., that it is an important health problem), (2) the screening tool (e.g., that it is safe, convenient and acceptable) and (3) the health care system (e.g., that effective treatment will be available for individuals who screen positive). These criteria should be met before service providers implement any screening program.

By far the most commonly used tool for screening for PPD is the Edinburgh Postnatal Depression Scale (EPDS). The Postpartum Depression Screening Scale (PDSS) is a more recent tool.

Research has not yet identified an optimal time to screen for PPD. If service providers are going to implement screening, they should determine the timing based on when, in their setting, they can reach the greatest number of new mothers.

Research has not yet answered the question of whether or not PPD screening can increase the number of women who will receive appropriate treatment, and ultimately recover from PPD. This is likely due to the high variability in the quality of care received by women identified with possible PPD.

Until further research takes place, we cannot strongly recommend implementing screening programs, since at present the potential costs outweigh the known benefits to mothers. However, health units and organizations with substantial economic and treatment resources may choose to be leaders in conducting the necessary research to examine the potential benefits of universal or targeted screening programs.

4
Prevention

What are preventive interventions?

What preventive interventions for postpartum depression have researchers and clinicians examined?

What can front-line service providers do to prevent postpartum depression in the mothers they work with?

Given the potentially serious long-term consequences of **postpartum depression** (PPD), researchers and clinicians have sought strategies for prevention. To date, the most common preventive strategy has been to modify a risk factor (Chapter 2) in order to decrease the likelihood of developing PPD (McLennan & Offord, 2002). For example, some researchers have provided women who have low levels of social support with additional support in the early postpartum period. However, translating risk factor research into effective preventive interventions has met with limited success. This is probably because PPD is a multifactorial illness, which likely has different causes, or triggers, in different women. As a result, it is unrealistic to expect that one single preventive strategy will work for all women.

More than 30 studies have evaluated prevention interventions for PPD, including pharmacological, psychological, psychosocial, educational and diverse models of care. While many of the researchers have provided sound theoretical reasons for the preventive approaches examined, most studies have design flaws, such as an insufficient number of participants or lack of an appropriate comparison group, and therefore provide insufficient evidence on which to base practice or policy recommendations (Dennis, 2004b; Dennis, 2004c). This chapter will review the research on the prevention of PPD, and will discuss potential strategies that front-line service providers may find helpful in their attempts to prevent PPD in the mothers they work with.

What Are Preventive Interventions?

THREE CATEGORIES OF PREVENTIVE INTERVENTIONS

Health professionals classify preventive interventions into the three categories below:

1. *Primary Prevention:* Primary prevention strategies include activities that aim to enhance protective factors and reduce the onset of particular problems. These activities target the general population, rather than simply a subgroup at risk. Primary prevention activities include immunization against disease, as well as the promotion of **self-care** activities among new mothers. Since successful primary prevention not only reduces but also prevents the suffering, cost and burden associated with disease, it is typically considered the most cost-effective form of health care.

2. *Secondary Prevention:* Secondary prevention efforts are more targeted toward specific subgroups expected to be at higher risk for particular problems, with the aim to interrupt or slow the progress of a condition by detecting and treating it early on. Secondary prevention interventions focus on early detection of common diseases that have significant risk for negative outcome without treatment. Screening tests for diseases such as hypertension, breast and prostate cancer are examples of secondary prevention activities: individuals who do not yet show symptoms of the disease undergo the screening tests. With early detection, service providers can often alter the course of the illness to maximize well-being and minimize suffering.

3. *Tertiary Prevention:* Tertiary prevention efforts slow the progress of a condition that is already established, with the aim to reduce disability that can result. These interventions aim specifically at preventing the progression of difficulties and complications.

   More information about preventive interventions appears in (Shah, 1998) and (Mrazek & Haggerty, 1994).

Preventive Interventions for PPD

Based on a comprehensive review (Dennis, 2004b; Dennis, 2004c), preventive interventions for PPD may be classified into the following approaches:

- psychosocial (e.g., enhancing social support systems)
- educational (e.g., providing additional information about PPD)
- improvements in quality of care (e.g., continuity of care)

- psychological (e.g., **cognitive-behavioural therapy** or **interpersonal psychotherapy**)
- pharmacological (e.g., antidepressants)
- hormonal (e.g., estrogen therapy).

Psychosocial Interventions

ANTENATAL AND POSTNATAL CLASSES

Pioneering work in the 1960s showed that realistic, solution-focused prenatal care could elevate women's postpartum mood and counter PPD (Gordon & Gordon, 1960). Based on this work, more recent trials have evaluated the preventive benefits of antenatal classes extending into the postpartum period (Brugha et al., 2000; Buist et al., 1999; Elliott et al., 2000; Stamp et al., 1995). Evidence from these international studies suggests that antenatal and postnatal classes with a focus on PPD have few preventive benefits, although the insignificant findings may partly reflect methodological problems with the studies (e.g., small sample sizes and failure of women enrolled in the trial to attend classes). More research is needed in this area to determine whether or not attending PPD-focused antenatal and postnatal classes is effective in preventing PPD.

INTRAPARTUM SUPPORT

Providing additional support during childbirth has also been examined as a strategy to prevent PPD. While two small trials evaluating the effect of **doula** support (continuous support during labour from an experienced laywoman) found mixed results, another trial that included more than 6,000 U.S. and Canadian women found that continuous labour support provided by a nurse had no protective effect against PPD (Hodnett et al., 2002). The results from this trial provide good evidence that continuous labour support cannot be recommended as a preventive strategy for PPD. However, intrapartum support may be beneficial for other maternal outcomes, such as decreased pain during labour.

HOME VISITS

To date, the efficacy of home visits provided by nurses in preventing PPD remains unknown. One well-designed study suggested that extensive home visits by nurses (weekly to six weeks, fortnightly to 12 weeks, and monthly to 24 weeks postpartum) prevented the development of PPD at six weeks postpartum; yet the protective effect was not maintained at 16 weeks, when rates of PPD were the same for mothers who received home visits as for those who did not (Armstrong et al., 1999; Armstrong et al., 2000). It is interesting to note that the 16-week assessment of PPD coincided with a decrease in intervention intensity of monthly home visits, raising the possibility that additional visits could have further maintained the positive effect.

It remains unclear whether or not support from a layperson is beneficial in preventing PPD. In a well-designed **randomized controlled trial**, the addition of home visits by a community support worker had no protective effect on the development of PPD (Morrell et al., 2000). However, a review of the lay support workers' activities in this trial revealed that the support workers spent more than 75 per cent of their time completing activities such as housework and infant care (specific types of instrumental support) and minimal time in providing emotional support to the mothers. This might have had a deleterious influence on the outcome of the study, since qualitative research suggests that women with PPD consistently describe a need to discuss emotional concerns, such as feelings of loneliness, worries about maternal competence, role conflicts and inability to cope (Chen et al., 1999; Nahas et al., 1999; Ritter et al., 2000; Small et al., 1994). Mothers with PPD considered instrumental support far less important than emotional support.

These studies suggest that additional research will have to determine whether or not home visits—either by a nurse, another service provider or a layperson—can prevent PPD, and if so, what the frequency, duration and content of the home visits should be.

POSTPARTUM SUPPORT GROUPS

Some research suggests that joining postpartum support groups might help to prevent PPD. However, as with the antenatal classes described above, poor and inconsistent postpartum group attendance rates pose a problem in the available research studies (Reid et al., 2002). Furthermore, some researchers have found a socio-economic bias among PPD group attendees, with "working class" mothers being less likely to attend group sessions than those who are more affluent (Reid et al., 2002).

Theoretically, postpartum support groups make sense as a possible preventive intervention in certain cultures, since they facilitate the sharing of new mothers' experiences and provide mother-to-mother peer support (Dennis, 2003a). Researchers will need to conduct further well-designed studies that address group attendance rates to provide evidence that support groups may help to prevent PPD. However, it is important to note that some cultures may discourage discussion of mental health issues, especially discussion outside of the family. While incorporating strategies that involve family members is critical for all mothers, it may be particularly salient for women from diverse cultures or those who live in rural or remote areas with limited health services.

Educational Interventions

The contribution of educational strategies in preventing PPD remains unclear. In one study, an educational package provided by a midwife informing women antenatally about PPD proved ineffective (Hayes et al., 2001). Yet in another study, advising mothers about available health service did help those who later developed PPD to seek appropriate treatment sooner (Okano et al., 1998).

This significant finding warrants further investigation: as described in Chapter 3, lack of knowledge about the existence and availability of health services is a key barrier to help-seeking that contributes to the underdetection of PPD. If researchers can show that educational or health promotion interventions consistently result in improved or faster access to treatment for women with PPD, these interventions may substantially reduce the burden of the illness for women and their families.

More research is needed to determine the effectiveness of educational interventions, as well as the content of such interventions.

Improving Quality of Care

Based on the idea that improving the quality of care provided to new mothers may influence maternal mood, diverse strategies have been examined, including continuity of care, early postpartum follow-up and flexible postpartum care.

CONTINUITY OF CARE

Since policy-makers have suggested that care that is more continuous and provided by the same health professional may increase women's satisfaction with perinatal services, new models of care now exist, including team midwifery. Two large trials have evaluated the impact of continuous midwifery-based care on diverse maternal outcomes and found no significant effects in preventing PPD. For these trials, team midwifery included a continuity of care model, where the same group of midwives followed women prenatally and into the postpartum period. Researchers need to conduct further studies to determine whether or not the results of these U.K. and Australian trials apply to Canada, with its different health care system.

EARLY POSTPARTUM FOLLOW-UP

Traditionally, health professionals have advised women to attend a six-week postpartum checkup with their primary health care provider. However, some researchers have hypothesized that earlier postpartum visits may either prevent or allow for the early identification and management of PPD. For example, one U.S. study examined the value of providing early communication in the immediate postpartum period (Serwint et al., 1991). In this trial, early communication consisted of a visit from the infant's future care provider 24 to 36 hours after delivery; special 24-hour telephone access to a physician, via a pager, for eight weeks; and a physician-initiated telephone call two to three days post-discharge to answer questions. Similarly, a **randomized controlled trial** investigated whether or not an earlier postpartum checkup visit to a **general practitioner** prevented the development of depressive symptoms and other negative health problems (Gunn et al., 1998). In this Australian trial, all participants received a letter and appointment date to visit a general practitioner for a checkup: the **intervention group** were given an appointment for one week after hospital discharge, the **control group** for six weeks postpartum. Neither of these studies found any evidence that follow-up care initiated sooner in the postpartum period prevented PPD.

FLEXIBLE POSTPARTUM CARE

Postpartum care tailored to the individual mother's needs shows some promise as a means of improving women's mental health and preventing PPD. Results from a large randomized controlled trial conducted in the United Kingdom showed that flexible, individualized midwifery-based care had a positive effect in preventing PPD (MacArthur et al., 2002). Since this well-conducted trial is one of the few to demonstrate significantly reduced rates of PPD, and as such to show potential for widespread implementation, a discussion of the intervention and its implications for the Canadian health care system follows in some detail here.

Midwives delivered the intervention by MacArthur and colleagues (2002). In the United Kingdom, midwives deliver most postnatal care, which includes visiting the new mother at home about seven times within the first two weeks postpartum. In this trial, the intervention group received extended midwifery care, such that the final home visit occurred at about four weeks postpartum, and the women's general practitioners saw and discharged them at 10 to 12 weeks postpartum. The content of the midwifery home visits was flexible, and could be tailored to the needs of each individual woman. To help in determining her needs, the participant was asked to complete a symptom checklist (including both physical and psychological symptoms) at the first visit, at days 10 and 28 postpartum, and at the discharge consultation. She also responded to the questions in the Edinburgh Postnatal Depression Scale (EPDS) on day 28 and at the discharge visit. MacArthur and colleagues developed evidence-based guidelines for assessment and referral to help midwives interpret the results of the symptom checklist and EPDS. For comparison, a control group received usual postpartum care from their midwives.

The effects of the intervention were assessed using self-report measures of physical and mental health, including the EPDS, which were administered by mail at four months postpartum. Results revealed that women who received the intervention had significantly lower EPDS scores than women who received usual postpartum care. In fact, in the intervention group, 14.4 per cent of participants had EPDS scores of 13 or more at four months postpartum, compared with

21.2 per cent of participants who received usual postpartum care. This difference was statistically significant, as were the differences between groups on the other mental health measures studied. No significant differences in physical health existed between the two groups (MacArthur et al., 2002).

Since the researchers designed the intervention to accommodate individual women's needs, it is impossible to determine which aspect or aspects of the intervention were responsible for the lower rates of PPD in the group of women who received extended care. Further research is needed to clarify this question. In addition, more than 14 per cent of women who received the supportive intervention still reported depressive symptoms. Given that 13 per cent of all new mothers experience PPD, care is needed in interpreting these study results. However, these results do provide the following preliminary evidence:

• Home visits by a service provider may reduce the risk of developing PPD, either by increasing the mother's social support, or by facilitating early detection and management of symptoms of depression. (See additional discussion of research on home visits on page 44.)
• Symptom checklists, including the EPDS, may also help to detect possible PPD.
• Tailoring postpartum care to the specific physical, emotional and social needs of the individual woman may be more effective in reducing the risk for PPD than are standardized protocols for postpartum care.

Given the significant differences between the U.K. and Canadian health care systems, a North American replication of MacArthur and colleagues' (2002) trial needs to take place before drawing any firm conclusions about the implications of flexible postpartum care in the prevention of PPD in Canadian women. However, the results of this important study give reason for optimism that effective strategies for the prevention of PPD will ultimately be available.

Psychological Interventions

INTERPERSONAL PSYCHOTHERAPY (IPT)

IPT was introduced as a time-limited, weekly outpatient treatment for depression provided by a specifically trained mental health professional (Klerman & Weissman, 1993). This approach focuses on the connection between the onset of depressive symptoms and possible interpersonal problems.

Researchers have conducted two studies to determine whether or not a preventive intervention based on the principles of IPT would reduce the risk of PPD. In one small pilot study, economically disadvantaged, high-risk women who attended group IPT sessions had fewer depressive symptoms at three months postpartum than did those who received routine care (Zlotnick et al., 2001). Another similar study evaluated 45 pregnant U.S. women with at least one PPD risk factor who received five individual IPT sessions, beginning in late pregnancy and ending at approximately four weeks postpartum (Gorman, 2001). Results from this small study also suggested that IPT may help prevent PPD.

The positive results from both these small studies indicate that additional research on the preventive efficacy of IPT is warranted. However, at present, accessibility to IPT is limited, since only specially trained mental health professionals (usually **psychiatrists**) can provide it, and any available resources are generally reserved to treat patients who have depression that is already established (rather than to prevent depression in women at risk). Therefore, in most communities, IPT is not a practical option for preventing PPD.

COGNITIVE-BEHAVIOURAL THERAPY (CBT)

Cognitive-behavioural therapy (CBT) is a strategy that has been successfully used to treat general depression. It is based on the notion that the way people perceive or think about an event determines in part how they will respond, including whether or not they will develop symptoms of depression (Hollon, 1998). According to **cognitive** theory, unhelpful beliefs about oneself underlie many mental health disorders. CBT aims to help people become more aware of how certain negative automatic thoughts, attitudes and beliefs contribute to their depression and how they can alter these thinking patterns so as to cope better.

To date, two trials (Chabrol et al., 2002; Saisto et al., 2001) have evaluated CBT as a means of preventing PPD. These trials provided conflicting and limited results, and further research is needed. However, like IPT, access to health care providers who are trained to administer CBT is limited in many areas. As a result, CBT is not available for PPD prevention in most communities.

PSYCHOLOGICAL DEBRIEFING

Health professionals and researchers have extensively debated the efficacy of "psychological debriefing" (a structured discussion with a trained health care provider about a critical life event) in recent years (Arendt & Elklit, 2001). Although its benefits are doubtful, researchers have tried debriefing as a strategy for preventing PPD. While one small U.K. study found that debriefing by a midwife may be helpful (Lavender & Walkinshaw, 1998), another large, well-conducted Australian trial involving women who had operative deliveries (e.g., Caesarean section, forceps delivery or vacuum extraction) showed that debriefing had a negative effect, increasing rather than decreasing emotional problems (Small et al., 2000); another large Australian study found no preventive effect (Priest et al., 2003). Thus, strong evidence suggests that psychological debriefing is *not* effective in preventing PPD, and it may be harmful.

Pharmacological Interventions

ANTIDEPRESSANT MEDICATION

Recent research suggests that the risk of depression recurring in women who have experienced PPD is as high as 40 per cent, with approximately 24 per cent of all recurrences happening within the first two weeks postpartum (Wisner et al., 2004). Women who have already experienced PPD are therefore understandably anxious about the depression recurring with any future births. For that reason, various studies have examined the **prophylactic** usefulness of antidepressants in preventing further episodes of PPD.

Research evidence to date shows mixed results in the recurrence of PPD for women who take prophylactic antidepressants. For example, in one small, well-conducted study with mothers who had previously experienced PPD, those who took the drug nortriptyline (Aventyl®) immediately after giving birth had no fewer recurrences than those who took a placebo (Wisner et al., 2001). Conversely, in another small study, mothers were randomly assigned to take sertraline (Zoloft®) (another type of antidepressant medication) or a placebo immediately after birth and were followed for 20 weeks postpartum (Wisner et al., 2004). Of 14 mothers who took sertraline, one (seven per cent) had a recurrence of the depression, while of the eight mothers who were assigned to take a placebo, four (50 per cent) had a recurrence. This difference was significant. These results suggest that the drug sertraline had more of a preventive effect than a placebo. While antidepressants may be advisable for women who are clinically depressed during pregnancy, their prophylactic use in women at risk for PPD is questionable and cannot be recommended at present.

Hormonal Interventions

Despite the sharp drop in circulating progesterone and estrogen immediately after birth, researchers have consistently failed to demonstrate a link between hormone levels and PPD (Harris, Johns et al., 1989; Harris et al., 1996). For example, O'Hara and colleagues (O'Hara et al., 1991) compared the hormone levels of child-bearing women who became depressed with the levels of those who did not. The researchers carried out frequent analyses of prolactin, progesterone, estradiol, free and total estriol, cortisol and urinary free cortisol during pregnancy and in the immediate postpartum, revealing few differences between those who had PPD and those who did not. However, other research has suggested that it may not be the levels of the hormones that are related to risk for PPD, but rather differences in individual sensitivity to hormone changes (Bloch et al., 2000). Several studies have examined the possibility of using hormone therapy to prevent PPD.

ESTROGEN THERAPY

In one U.S. study where seven women with a history of mood disorders received high-dose oral estrogen immediately following delivery, only one became depressed and needed treatment with psychotropic medications within the first year postpartum (Sichel et al., 1995). The low rate of relapse in this small study suggests a need for further research on the prophylactic ability of estrogen to prevent postpartum mood disorders from recurring in mothers known to be at risk. However, health professionals must address both efficacy and safety issues associated with the use of estrogen before estrogen therapy can be routinely recommended for use in perinatal women.

PROGESTERONE THERAPY

The prophylactic use of progesterone for PPD has been frequently proposed (Dalton, 1976; Dalton, 1994). However, there has only been one randomized controlled trial conducted to determine the effect of a single dose of progestogen (norethisterone enanthate) administered postnatally on PPD. In this study, researchers found an increase in depressive symptoms at six weeks postpartum among women given the progesterone (Lawrie et al., 1998). This evidence indicates that progesterone therapies *should not* be used in the immediate postpartum period.

THYROID HORMONE THERAPY

Research suggests that women who are positive for thyroid antibodies during pregnancy are at increased risk of developing PPD (Harris, Fung et al., 1989; Pop et al., 1993). To test the hypothesis that stabilizing postpartum thyroid function by daily thyroxine administration might reduce the onset and severity of depression, researchers conducted a randomized controlled trial in the United Kingdom (Harris et al., 2002). This well-conducted trial found no evidence that thyroxine decreases the occurrence of PPD, and the researchers suggested that known risk factors, such as negative life events, more likely trigger the higher rate of PPD in thyroid-antibody–positive women than does abnormal thyroid function.

What Can Service Providers Do?

HOW CAN SERVICE PROVIDERS HELP PREVENT PPD?

While it is true that the research evidence has not yet identified any single strategy that can consistently prevent PPD in all women, this is in part due to methodological problems in the research (e.g., small sample sizes, high drop-out rates). It is unlikely that any one standardized prevention strategy will effectively prevent PPD in all women, considering the complexity of this multifactorial condition.

However, this does not mean that nothing can be done to reduce the negative effects of PPD on women and their families. Future research studies are likely to confirm some of the promising preliminary results described in this chapter, and to elucidate additional strategies for prevention, which have not yet been tested.

Recently, one of the authors completed a Cochrane systematic review to examine the effectiveness of preventive psychosocial or psychological interventions (Dennis & Creedy, 2004). When data from methodologically strong randomized controlled trials were combined and analysed using meta-analysis, some trends emerged that may help to explain which types of preventive interventions are more likely to effectively reduce rates of PPD. On the basis of the available evidence, the following factors appear to be associated with more successful preventive strategies. The intervention:

- is administered to women identified as being "at risk" for PPD, rather than to the total population of pregnant or postpartum women
- occurs during the postpartum period, rather than the antenatal period
- is individually based, rather than group-based.

Further research is needed to evaluate the effectiveness of interventions that incorporate these factors. However, the results from this meta-analysis suggest that providing individually tailored postpartum care to women identified as being at risk for PPD may reduce rates of PPD. As health units and organizations work toward the goal of providing holistic, multidisciplinary care to perinatal women, they may find some of the strategies described in this chapter to be beneficial.

Summary

Preventive interventions are strategies that aim to reduce the negative effects of PPD, either by stopping it from developing (primary prevention) or facilitating early detection and treatment (secondary and tertiary prevention).

Researchers and clinicians have evaluated various PPD prevention strategies, including antidepressants, psychotherapy, additional support and hormonal therapy.

To date, no prevention strategy has been consistently found to prevent PPD, and researchers urgently need to conduct more studies in this area. However, interventions are more likely to have a preventive effect if they target "at-risk" women, are initiated during the postnatal period and are individually based.

5
Treatment

Does postpartum depression require treatment?

What treatments are likely to be effective for postpartum depression?

Are antidepressants safe for use while breastfeeding?

Seventy to 80 per cent of women with **postpartum depression** (PPD) are successfully treated and recover. Treatment of PPD is generally the same as that for depression that occurs at any other time in a woman's life. While mild to moderate PPD may respond to psychotherapy or social interventions, severe episodes usually require antidepressants in addition to support and therapy. Once a health professional has identified major depression, the mother and her caregivers must recognize it as a serious illness that requires treatment.

PPD, especially if prolonged and untreated, is detrimental to the mother's health, and can disrupt family relationships, undermine infant-mother attachment and possibly impair the child's long-term development (see Chapter 7). In fact, just identifying and acknowledging PPD as a potentially serious disorder and discussing possible therapies can be a first step. It may help the mother who is depressed in easing her uncertainty about what is wrong with her, and in helping to dispel fears that she is a failure, inadequate or "going crazy."

Current Options for Treating PPD

For mild to moderate episodes of PPD, psychotherapy, counselling and increased support (e.g., attendance at peer support groups, more help from partner and family) may help to alleviate the depressed mood. However, severe PPD usually requires treatment with antidepressants, often along with some form of psychotherapy (Stewart et al., 2003).

TREATMENTS FOR PPD

A comprehensive review of the literature revealed a wide range of treatments for PPD (Dennis, 2004d; Dennis & Stewart, 2004). These include:

- antidepressants (good evidence for effectiveness in depression in general)
- psychotherapy, such as **interpersonal** or **cognitive-behavioural therapy** (good evidence for effectiveness in depression in general)
- supportive counselling (more research evidence needed)
- increased social support—from friends, relatives, peers (e.g., support groups) (more research evidence needed)
- more emotional and practical support from the mother's partner or spouse, and others (more research evidence needed)
- electroconvulsive therapy, or ECT (for severe or unresponsive depression) (good evidence for effectiveness in depression in general)
- maternal relaxation/massage therapy for mild depression (more research evidence needed)
- hormone (estrogen) therapy (still experimental)
- bright light therapy (still experimental).

Making Informed, Evidence-Based Decisions about PPD Treatment

Although untreated PPD typically remits in seven to 12 months, a woman with PPD should receive treatment to hasten recovery, prevent harmful consequences and diminish the likelihood of relapses (Wisner et al., 2002). Prompt treatment can not only shorten the duration of PPD and lessen the mother's distress, but also may prevent marital and family discord, and lessen the impact on children.

Quite frequently, not only mothers who are depressed but also health professionals fail to recognize or acknowledge the fact that major depression does not merely entail low mood (feeling sad, anxious and worried), but is also a serious condition that requires treatment. Simply offering reassurance and psychosocial support is not sufficient to manage PPD.

Service providers can help women who are depressed by encouraging them to express their feelings and misgivings. Providers can also dispel misleading and idealized notions of motherhood, and replace these myths with a more practical and realistic picture of parenthood (see Chapter 9). In addition, they can provide women with PPD with accurate, specific information about what, where and how to access specialized mental health care services.

Current evidence suggests that although psychotherapy and increased social and practical support may be enough to diminish mild PPD, more severe episodes usually require the use of antidepressants, in addition to therapy and support, to recover and stay well. While good scientific evidence confirms the usefulness of antidepressants in reducing depression that occurs at other times in life, less research exists about their specific use during the postpartum period (Appleby et al., 1997).

Given the uncertainty about the best way to treat PPD in individual women, the mother and her health care providers must weigh the latest evidence for the benefits versus risks of any treatment and jointly decide which to choose based on her needs. In selecting therapy, the mother must consider not only the effects of depression on herself, but also its impact on others in her family. The consequences of PPD may be worse when there are other adverse circumstances, such as marital or relationship discord, poverty and lack of support (Murray & Cooper, 1997).

Evaluating Antidepressants Used for PPD

There are now many antidepressants to treat major depression. Generally, a **family physician** or **psychiatrist** prescribes these medications. (For information about antidepressant dosages, see Appendix C, page 155.)

To date, there are no official "guidelines" for the professional management of PPD. However, there are published "consensus statements" based on expert opinions. These statements include suggestions for how long women should take these drugs to maintain recovery and for their use while breastfeeding (Altshuler et al., 2001).

Please note that the generic names of the following antidepressants appear alphabetically.

FREQUENTLY PRESCRIBED ANTIDEPRESSANTS

The antidepressants most frequently prescribed to treat PPD are the selective serotonin reuptake inhibitors (SSRIs) and the newer serotonin-norepinephrine reuptake inhibitors (SNRIs). The SSRIs include:
- citalopram (Celexa®)
- fluoxetine (Prozac®)
- fluvoxamine (Luvox®)
- sertraline (Zoloft®).

SNRIs include:
- duloxetine (Cymbalta®)
- venlafaxine (Effexor®).

OLDER MEDICATIONS

Clinicians still sometimes prescribe older medications, such as the tricyclic antidepressants (TCAs), for women with PPD despite the fact that these medications are more likely to produce unpleasant side-effects. However, they are also more effective for some women.

The tricyclic antidepressants include:
- amitriptyline (Elavil®)
- clomipramine (Anafranil®)
- desipramine (Norpramin®)
- doxepin (Sinequan®)
- imipramine (Tofranil®)
- nortriptyline (Aventyl®)
- trimipramine (Surmontil®).

"ATYPICAL" ANTIDEPRESSANTS

Health providers may also suggest another class of medications, called the "atypical" antidepressants (because they don't fit neatly into the other drug classes), for women with PPD. They include:
- bupropion (Wellbutrin®)
- mirtazapine (Remeron®)
- moclobemide (Manerix®)
- phenelzine (Nardil®).

SIDE-EFFECTS

Common side-effects (usually transient) of antidepressants include:
- appetite loss, nausea, diarrhea or constipation
- dry mouth
- sweating
- agitation, insomnia
- sleepiness, fatigue
- weight gain (with some of them)
- decreased libido (with some of them)
- headaches.

Many of these side-effects disappear within two to three weeks, but if they are severe and don't disappear, women should discuss the side-effects with the treating physician. Since women who have recently given birth may be especially sensitive to medications, some experts suggest that antidepressant therapy be initiated at half the usual starting dose for depression (e.g., 25 mg of sertraline per day, or 10 mg paroxetine daily) for four days, then gradually increased by small increments (Wisner et al., 2002). It usually takes a few weeks before antidepressants produce a noticeable mood improvement. For example, while some mothers who are depressed show signs of clinical improvement within one to two weeks of starting antidepressants, others may take up to six weeks to feel better. Sometimes it is necessary to alter the drug dose or switch to another medication before improvement occurs, but this should usually only happen after several weeks of therapy, and in consultation with the woman's physician.

For a first bout of depression, the woman should continue the medication for at least six months after achieving remission to prevent relapse. A woman on antidepressants should not stop taking the medications suddenly, but should gradually taper her dose to prevent withdrawal symptoms, always in consultation with her physician. Sudden withdrawal of antidepressants can cause flu-like symptoms, dizziness and nightmares.

Anxiety may accompany PPD, and may initially increase with antidepressants. As a result, some women are prescribed minor tranquilizers (such as clonazepam [Rivotril®], diazepam [Valium®] or lorazepam [Ativan®]) to diminish their anxiety. They should use the tranquilizers for only a limited time (i.e., only until the antidepressants begin to work) to minimize risks of dependency (Robinson & Stewart, 2001).

Use of Antidepressants While Breastfeeding

Breastfeeding has significant health benefits for the infant and is psychologically important to many mothers. Mothers who wish to breastfeed may be reluctant to take antidepressants or other medications for fear of the possible effects on the baby of exposure to small amounts of the drug transmitted through breast milk. In such cases, service providers must weigh the mother's objections to using antidepressants against the detrimental effects of depression (Newport et al., 2002).

Controversy continues about the effects of psychotropic medications on breastfeeding infants (Stewart, 2000; Hendrick et al., 2003; Weissman et al., 2004). Most antidepressant medications and their metabolites pass into breast milk (although the amounts are small and highly variable), so mothers who need antidepressants are sometimes advised to wait eight or nine hours after taking antidepressants before breastfeeding. This will require pumping milk and refrigerating it during the time of day when antidepressant levels are low to use in feeding during the eight hours after taking antidepressants. The plasma of most nursing infants whose mothers are taking antidepressants also contains small detectable levels of some antidepressants. For this reason, health providers should monitor young babies of these breastfeeding mothers to assess for any ill effects in the baby, such as jitteriness, sleepiness or poor sucking ability.

Overall, it appears to be relatively safe for mothers who are depressed to take the medications commonly used for severe PPD—including SSRIs, such as sertraline (Zoloft) and paroxetine (Paxil), and TCAs, such as nortriptyline (Aventyl)—while breastfeeding full-term, healthy babies (Stewart, 2000; Wisner et al., 2002; Weissman et al., 2004). There is less evidence about the effects of a breastfeeding mother's antidepressant use in premature infants, or for use of newer antidepressants (such as mirtazapine [Remeron], bupropion [Wellbutrin] or moclobemide [Manerix]).

Researchers have not completed any well-designed, randomized controlled studies on the effect of antidepressants in the infants of breastfeeding mothers, and there are no evidence-based guidelines for their use during lactation (Stewart, 2000; Weissman et al., 2004). Recent research and a Health Canada warning caution women and their physicians to carefully consider the use of antidepressants during pregnancy—especially shortly before birth (Laine et al., 2003; Zeskind & Stephens, 2004; Ross et al., in press). This new research and warning suggest that the effects of the much smaller amounts of antidepressants present in breast milk should also be studied in infants. The American Academy of Pediatrics Committee on Drugs (2001) states that mothers who take antidepressants may continue breastfeeding (if they wish to do so), provided health professionals monitor the infants for possible side-effects. As the brain's neurotransmitter system continues to develop in infants after birth, the long-term effects of antidepressant drugs on young children remain unknown. Since many antidepressants have only recently come onto the market, there are still no published studies about their long-term effects in children exposed to them through breast milk.

In the final analysis, the mother and her physician (and perhaps also her partner, if she has one) must weigh the potential risks of infant exposure to medications through breast milk against the possibly serious consequences of the mother's untreated depression, and jointly decide which feeding method is the best choice for her and her baby. Ultimately, the goal is to treat the depression in a timely fashion.

Psychotherapy as a Treatment for PPD

Psychotherapies, such as interpersonal psychotherapy (IPT) or cognitive-behavioural therapy (CBT), can be effective in alleviating mild to moderate PPD. As many women are unwilling to take medication while pregnant or breastfeeding (Chabrol et al., 2004), psychotherapy may be a successful alternative or may serve as a first-line therapy. However, many of these therapies require specially trained practitioners, and so may be difficult to access. Long-term outcomes (e.g., beyond the first few weeks or months of treatment) of these therapies are still unknown.

INTERPERSONAL PSYCHOTHERAPY (IPT)

IPT focuses on the changing roles of parenthood and improving relationship dynamics. It has proven effective in reducing depressive symptoms and improving social function in women with PPD. IPT can also help to resolve the marital or relationship conflicts that are common among new parents (Stuart & O'Hara, 1995). Provided they have had the appropriate training, psychiatrists, **psychologists**, nurses or social workers may offer this form of psychotherapy. Preliminary studies with group IPT also show positive results in treating PPD. However, further research is needed to confirm the long-term benefits of IPT in new mothers.

COGNITIVE-BEHAVIOURAL THERAPY (CBT)

CBT aims to replace negative thought patterns with a more reality-based and positive **cognitive** style that improves coping skills. CBT is commonly used to treat mild to moderate depression. Several small studies have shown CBT to be useful in reducing depressive symptoms and hastening recovery from PPD. (For a fuller description of CBT, see page 46 in Chapter 4.)

PSYCHODYNAMIC PSYCHOTHERAPY

Psychodynamic psychotherapy is an analytical approach that probes the unconscious and conscious roots of feelings and behaviour. One study found that this method has only short-term remedial benefits in easing the depressive symptoms of PPD and, in the long run, appears to be no better than spontaneous remission (Cooper et al., 2003; Murray et al., 2003). More studies are needed to evaluate this type of psychotherapy.

PEER SUPPORT GROUPS

Many studies confirm that lack of support is a strong risk factor for the development of PPD. The frequently voiced complaints of women with PPD include:
• having no one who understands them or with whom they can talk openly
• thinking no other mothers feel as bad as they do, and that the others are not failures
• lacking an intimate friend/partner/confidante with whom to share feelings
• receiving no support without specifically asking for it
• lacking peer companionship (interacting with other new mothers).

Some women describe the positive effects of attending a peer support group—how it creates hope by allowing them to identify with other women in similar situations, normalizing their experiences, and demonstrating that others share their feelings.

However, studies investigating the efficacy of group sessions (run by psychologists, nurses or occupational therapists) in alleviating PPD have shown conflicting results. Some support groups did apparently improve maternal mood (as measured by the **Edinburgh Postnatal Depression Scale** [EPDS]); others had no effect. Therefore, while some peer support and professionally led therapy groups for mothers who are depressed appear to help in alleviating PPD, researchers need to work further to demonstrate which types of group therapy, group dynamics and leadership are most effective.

It is difficult for mothers with a new baby to get out regularly to attend group meetings. As a result, some women have participated in a trial with telephone-based peer support, provided by mothers who had previously experienced PPD: this method shows promise in improving maternal mood (Dennis, 2003a). A larger, multi-site trial evaluating the effect of telephone-based peer support is currently being conducted by Dr. Dennis in the Toronto area.

NON-DIRECTIVE COUNSELLING

According to two small European trials, non-directive counselling, or "listening home visits," given by nurses, social workers, health visitors or psychologists, appear to have a positive impact in reducing the depressive symptoms of PPD. However, a large randomized trial is needed to replicate these results.

Hormone Therapy

Some researchers and clinicians have advocated estrogen therapy as a treatment for PPD. Preliminary results from small studies evaluating the use of 17 beta-estradiol, given either as tablets under the tongue or as a skin patch, found the depressive symptoms of PPD were significantly reduced (Gregoire et al., 1996; Ahokas et al., 2001; Karuppaswamy & Vlies, 2003). However, in some of the studies where estrogen therapy diminished the women's depression, the women were also taking antidepressants, confounding the results. Given the flaws of the studies done so far, further research is needed to confirm the efficacy of estrogen in alleviating PPD, the safest dose to use, its possible side-effects (such as blood clots), as well as its effects on the infant if taken while breastfeeding.

Women with PPD should not take progesterone or progestogens (which are in certain contraceptives) as these compounds may increase depression.

Electroconvulsive Therapy (ECT)

ECT consists of briefly applying an electric current to the brain while the person is anesthetized. There is little research evidence available to guide practitioners in the use of ECT for women with PPD. However, in clinical settings, clinicians use ECT for severe depression with good results, and they consider it as safe for use in postpartum women as it is for general use. ECT would seldom serve as a first-line therapy for PPD, unless the woman is acutely suicidal or infanticidal, but it can be a valuable clinical tool for mothers who are severely depressed who do not respond to or do not wish to take antidepressants; this is particularly so because people often respond very quickly to ECT (Robinson & Stewart, 2001).

Bright Light Therapy

A few small studies suggest that bright light therapy (still experimental for PPD) might have an antidepressant effect, and might perhaps be a viable alternative for mothers who are depressed who do not respond to, or do not wish to accept, traditional approaches (Epperson et al., 2004). More studies are needed.

Complementary or Alternative Therapies

Complementary or alternative therapies for PPD include massage therapy, acupuncture, herbal remedies (such as St. John's wort, black cohosh), dietary supplements and aromatherapy (Weier & Beal, 2004). However, there is no research evidence to indicate that these therapies are effective.

Some women, in particular those who breastfeed their infants, may prefer to try natural therapies rather than traditional medical treatments such as antidepressants. However, women must remember that natural therapies can also have side-effects and may interact with other medications that a new mother might be taking. In addition, just as antidepressants pass into the mother's breast milk, any herbal or naturopathic substances that a lactating mother takes will do likewise. Women should therefore check with their doctors to ensure that any substances they plan to ingest, including herbal remedies, are safe for themselves and/or their baby. Moreover, many herbal remedies, such as St. John's wort, can have serious interactions with other medications. There is often no reliable information available about the safety of many herbal remedies, and their purity and strength often vary from sample to sample.

RELAXATION OR MASSAGE THERAPY

A few small studies have shown that massage and relaxation exercises for mothers with depression can elevate mood and decrease anxiety, and can be useful in countering mild depression. Despite some promising early results, the usefulness of massage and/or relaxation in relieving mild PPD remains uncertain due to conflicting outcomes of studies.

Summary

PPD is a serious illness that requires treatment. If prolonged and untreated, PPD can negatively affect the health of mother, baby and the entire family.

Treatment options for PPD should be chosen based on the woman's needs and preference, the severity of her symptoms and the availability of services. The most common forms of treatment for PPD are:

- psychotherapy (especially CBT and IPT)
- antidepressants
- peer support groups and social support as an adjunct to antidepressants and psychotherapy.

Current evidence suggests that commonly prescribed antidepressants (e.g., sertraline, paroxetine and nortriptyline) are probably safe for mothers to use when breastfeeding healthy, full-term infants. However, there are no long-term outcome studies. Whether or not a mother decides to take antidepressants while breastfeeding requires careful evaluation of the risks versus benefits of treatment for herself and her infant.

The overriding goal should be the prompt treatment of the depression.

6

Making Referrals for Assessment and Treatment

When should a service provider refer a woman for postpartum depression assessment and/or treatment?

Where or to whom should she be referred?

Often, a primary role of the front-line health care worker is to refer women with suspected **postpartum depression** (PPD) for further assessment and/or treatment. This chapter will provide information about when referral is necessary and to whom referrals should be made. In addition, the chapter explains what roles various health care and social services can play in the assessment and treatment of PPD, as well as how women can access these providers and services.

When Should Service Providers Make a Referral?

A referral for assessment of potential PPD should be considered whenever a mother, her family and/or her service provider is concerned about her mood or behaviour. These concerns may arise in many ways:

- The mother may spontaneously report that she is feeling depressed, sad or worried; she may complain about physical symptoms such as no appetite, inability to sleep and/or extreme fatigue; or she may simply state that she hasn't been feeling like herself.

- The woman's partner or other family members may report that she has seemed depressed or has complained of the symptoms described above and in Chapter 1. (See page 5.)
- A mother may score above an established threshold on a screening tool such as the **Edinburgh Postnatal Depression Scale**, or EPDS. (See Chapter 3, page 30.)
- Based on clinical experience or familiarity with the woman, her service provider may notice a change from the woman's usual self or symptoms that are consistent with a possible diagnosis of PPD.

As described in Chapter 1, women experience a range of emotions during the postpartum period, and transient feelings of sadness or worry do not necessarily indicate PPD. However, a health professional should always assess severe mood changes, particularly if they appear suddenly. Figure 6–1 provides some guidelines for determining when a mother's symptoms fall outside of the normal range, and therefore warrant referral for further assessment.

However, what appear to be "normal" mood changes can sometimes mask PPD in its early stages. For this reason, the service provider should carefully follow any woman who reports symptoms of depression. As discussed in Chapter 1, a diagnosis of PPD requires that symptoms be present for two or more weeks. Therefore, whenever you decide not to refer, you should follow the woman as often as necessary over several weeks to ensure that the symptoms have not persisted or worsened into an episode of PPD.

Figure 6–1 (see page 63) provides a guideline only. The clinical impression and expertise of the service provider should be an important component of decision-making. When in doubt, err on the side of caution: it is better to make an unnecessary referral than to miss referring someone who is in need of treatment.

EMERGENCY PSYCHIATRIC REFERRALS: THOUGHTS OF SUICIDE/INFANTICIDE

Figure 6–1 demonstrates that symptoms of **psychosis** (see Chapter 1) and thoughts of self-harm warrant emergency psychiatric referral: that is, a **psychiatrist** should assess the mother as soon as possible, and certainly within 24 hours. The mother should not be alone (by herself or with the baby) until the assessment has taken place.

Individual health units and agencies may have different policies about how to handle emergency psychiatric referrals. Service providers should discuss these policies with their managers, preferably before the need for them arises. In most situations, an emergency psychiatric referral will involve accompanying the mother to the nearest hospital emergency department, where the psychiatrist on call or the emergency physician will assess her and admit her if necessary. If the woman already has an established relationship with a psychiatrist, she may have received emergency contact information. In this case, the emergency referral can be made to her own psychiatrist (so long as this person is able to see her within 24 hours).

FIGURE 6–1

Decision Tree for Assessment and Referral of Women with Possible PPD

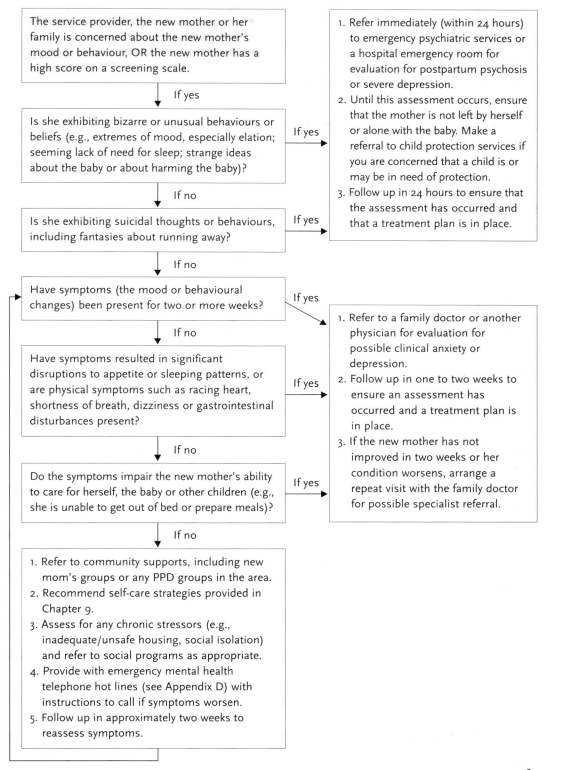

The service provider, the new mother or her family is concerned about the new mother's mood or behaviour, OR the new mother has a high score on a screening scale.

If yes

Is she exhibiting bizarre or unusual behaviours or beliefs (e.g., extremes of mood, especially elation; seeming lack of need for sleep; strange ideas about the baby or about harming the baby)?

If no

Is she exhibiting suicidal thoughts or behaviours, including fantasies about running away?

If no

Have symptoms (the mood or behavioural changes) been present for two or more weeks?

If no

Have symptoms resulted in significant disruptions to appetite or sleeping patterns, or are physical symptoms such as racing heart, shortness of breath, dizziness or gastrointestinal disturbances present?

If no

Do the symptoms impair the new mother's ability to care for herself, the baby or other children (e.g., she is unable to get out of bed or prepare meals)?

If no

If yes →

If yes →

1. Refer immediately (within 24 hours) to emergency psychiatric services or a hospital emergency room for evaluation for postpartum psychosis or severe depression.
2. Until this assessment occurs, ensure that the mother is not left by herself or alone with the baby. Make a referral to child protection services if you are concerned that a child is or may be in need of protection.
3. Follow up in 24 hours to ensure that the assessment has occurred and that a treatment plan is in place.

If yes →

If yes →

If yes →

1. Refer to a family doctor or another physician for evaluation for possible clinical anxiety or depression.
2. Follow up in one to two weeks to ensure an assessment has occurred and a treatment plan is in place.
3. If the new mother has not improved in two weeks or her condition worsens, arrange a repeat visit with the family doctor for possible specialist referral.

1. Refer to community supports, including new mom's groups or any PPD groups in the area.
2. Recommend self-care strategies provided in Chapter 9.
3. Assess for any chronic stressors (e.g., inadequate/unsafe housing, social isolation) and refer to social programs as appropriate.
4. Provide with emergency mental health telephone hot lines (see Appendix D) with instructions to call if symptoms worsen.
5. Follow up in approximately two weeks to reassess symptoms.

In some regions, it may not be possible to arrange for a psychiatric assessment within 24 hours. In these cases, the emergency referral should be made to another physician in the same region who has some mental health expertise. Information about arranging for psychiatric consultations in underserviced regions appears on page 73.

Suicidal ideation

A mother who is depressed may say things signifying thoughts of harming herself and/or her baby, with phrases such as, "It might be best to end it all," or, "My baby would be better off without me." A woman with suicidal thoughts is likely to score greater than zero on item 10 of the EPDS (see Chapter 3).

Each department or organization may have specific protocols in place to address suicide risk. In the absence of these types of protocols, however, it can sometimes be it difficult to establish whether or not a new mother is truly suicidal, or whether she is simply expressing her feelings of being overwhelmed and frustrated.

A front-line service provider can ask the following questions* to help determine whether or not an emergency referral is necessary:

- How often do you have thoughts of harming yourself?
- How severe are these feelings? / How much have they been bothering you?
- Have you had these kinds of feelings before? If so, what happened? / How did you cope with them?
- Have you made any previous suicide/self-harm attempts?
- Have you thought about how you would harm yourself?
- What support do you currently have at home?
- [If she has a partner] Have you talked about how you are feeling with him/her?
- Are you close to your parents/other family members? Do they know how you have been feeling?
- Can you count on your partner and/or family to give you emotional support?
- [If she does not have a partner or family members available to give support] Is there anyone else in your life whose support you can call on?
- Have you told this person or anyone else about your feelings?
- Could you phone this person and would he/she come if you felt you needed support?

---

* Adapted with permission from Holden, 1994.

> **Immediate emergency psychiatric referral is essential if the mother has:**
> • frequent suicidal thoughts or is overwhelmed by thoughts of suicide
> OR IF
> • she has a plan and means
> OR IF
> • she has no reliable support.
>   The mother should not be left by herself or alone with the baby until she is assessed.

In cases where an emergency psychiatric referral is not needed (or is not immediately available), the front-line service provider or the woman's **family physician** needs to follow up carefully to ensure that symptoms do not worsen. As stated above, it is always best to err on the side of caution when suicide is a concern.

Thoughts of harming the infant

Thoughts of harming the infant are common in PPD, and usually take the form of fleeting mental pictures that pop into the woman's head without warning: she may see herself wilfully hurting the baby (e.g., drowning the baby while bathing, throwing the baby off a bridge, pushing the stroller into traffic, cutting the baby with a kitchen knife).

Although these thoughts are often scary and distressing, they seldom indicate that she will actually harm her child. In fact, a recent study of mothers and fathers of new babies found that 65 per cent of parents reported such thoughts (Abramowitz et al., 2003). In most cases, they are probably a normal reaction to the intense vigilance new parents feel in the context of the responsibility of caring for a baby.

Of course, these scary thoughts require clinical attention if:
• the mother thinks the thoughts are reasonable, or that she may act on them
• the mother finds she cannot put the thoughts out of her head or is constantly worrying about when the next scary thought will come
• the thoughts are troublesome enough that the mother is taking action to avoid hurting her baby (e.g., putting away all the knives and sharp objects; refusing to leave the house)
• **suicidal ideation** or psychotic symptoms accompany the thoughts.

In these cases, the service provider should make an emergency psychiatric referral, as described above.

In cases of fleeting scary thoughts where suicide and psychosis are not a concern, the mother can be reassured that although they are frightening, these thoughts are quite normal: it is exceedingly rare for these women to harm their infants, except in the context of severe suicidal ideation or psychotic symptoms as described above. As for all women with PPD, the front-line service provider or the woman's family physician needs to follow up to watch for worsening symptoms or developing suicidal ideation.

Referrals to Child Protection Services

In working with postpartum women, occasions may arise when you are concerned about the possibility of child abuse or neglect. As a result, you need to be familiar with the applicable reporting legislation.

Child protection is provincially regulated, so the wording of reporting obligations varies between provinces and territories. In Ontario, the *Child and Family Services Act* states: "If a person has reasonable grounds to suspect that a child is or may be in need of protection, the person must promptly report the suspicion and the information upon which it is based to a Children's Aid Society." (See www.children.gov.on.ca/CS/en/programs/ChildProtection/Publications/ repChAbuse.htm.)

The responsibility to report is similar in other provinces and territories, and information about the regulations that apply is available from each local child protection agency.

Most of the regulations include subjective terms such as "reasonable grounds." This means that service providers will need to use their judgment as to whether or not there is reason to suspect that a child needs protection. For example, does the care provider/parent have the necessary physical, mental and emotional capacity and/or support to provide care to the child? If the child is or may be in need of protection, service providers have a duty to report their concerns directly to a child protection agency as soon as these concerns are identified. You should consult with child protection services if there is any uncertainty as to whether or not a referral is necessary.

Service providers must carefully document details of their concerns, any referral and/or consultation with the child protection agency, and any follow-up intervention identified by the child protection agency (if it is disclosed to them). In most cases, women with postpartum psychiatric disorders do not pose a risk to their children, as long as the mothers receive prompt and appropriate treatment and support. However, in mothers who are severely mentally ill, risk of harm to or neglect of a child may be a reality. If this suspicion arises, the risk must be reported to child protection services. For this reason, all service providers who come into contact with children should be alert for warning signs of child abuse and neglect.

Where Should Service Providers Refer a Mother Who May Have PPD?

To whom service providers refer the mother depends on the nature and severity of the symptoms the woman is experiencing, availability/accessibility of services in the area and the woman's own preferences. Figure 6–1 provides recommendations based on symptom severity and persistence.

INVOLVING THE MOTHER IN REFERRAL DECISIONS

Whenever possible, include the mother (and her partner and/or family members, if appropriate) as an active participant in deciding whether or not and where to refer. Being inclusive will ensure that she is as invested as possible in following through with the recommendations for her care.

Before making a referral, explain to the new mother why you feel it is necessary (e.g., she is showing symptoms of PPD; you are concerned about her suicidal feelings) and what she can expect to get out of a referral (e.g., she will be able to see a doctor who can assess her symptoms and recommend a treatment plan; she will have the opportunity to attend a support group and meet other women who are dealing with similar issues). Present the various options for treatment and inquire about the new mother's preferences and past experiences.

You should also investigate potential referral sources before recommending them to the mother. Your agency or organization may have specific criteria for identifying appropriate referral sources. You may find it helpful to generate a list of referral sources that others have had good experiences with. Check out the training, credentials and regulation of any individuals you are considering. Be aware of the preferences and philosophies of the health care professionals and organizations you are referring to. Do the professionals and organizations endorse a biomedical or **biopsychosocial model** of PPD? Do they support women's decisions about treatment? Knowing as much as possible about referral sources will help women make informed choices about where to go for help. Unfortunately, many service providers have limited knowledge about PPD, and as a result, may dismiss or ignore women's concerns about their mood. Front-line service providers can play an important role as advocates for women with their physicians.

Here are some suggestions to help the mother prepare for her appointment with the physician:

• If the referral is to a family physician, tell the receptionist who books the appointment the purpose of the visit (so long as the woman consents to this). Otherwise, the receptionist will book the standard (very short) time slot, and the woman may have to return for a second visit.

- Coach the mother as to how best to present her concerns to the physician: describe concrete examples, such as "I have only been sleeping for three hours each night because I am awake worrying about the baby" or "I am feeling so miserable that I have lost my appetite and haven't eaten a proper meal in a week." It is also important for the mother to tell the physician how long the symptoms have been present, and how they have been affecting her ability to care for herself and the baby.
- Encourage the mother to write down a list of questions and requests to take into the office with her. In her state of distress or anxiety, she may forget to tell the doctor important information.
- Encourage the woman to bring her partner or another supportive person to the appointment with her, since she may find it difficult to remember to ask all of her questions or retain all of the information the physician gives her.
- Consider preparing a letter signed by you that the woman can take with her to the physician, detailing her specific symptoms and how long those symptoms have been present. If you have administered the EPDS or another screening tool to the woman, you might want to enclose a copy of the results (with the consent of the mother). Letting the physician know that another health care or social service provider has found the woman's symptoms to be a concern may encourage him or her to take them seriously.

Always follow up with the mother to ensure that she met with the health care provider you referred her to, and that an appropriate treatment plan has been established.

The process of accessing care for mental health issues can be frightening and overwhelming at the best of times—even more so when women are trying to juggle their own needs with those of a new infant. Women may be much more likely to follow through with your recommendations if they feel assured that in developing the referral plan, you have carefully considered their best interests, as well as the best interests of their families.

WHAT IF THE MOTHER REFUSES THE REFERRAL?

Despite your best intentions, you may encounter situations in which a mother refuses any referrals or support. Unfortunately, this situation is not uncommon among women who report suicidal thoughts and/or symptoms of psychosis.

A woman must almost always consent before a service provider can share information about her symptoms and/or situation with someone else, including other service providers or her family members (see exceptions to this in the following paragraph). If she does not consent to see another health professional and/or agree that you can discuss her situation with another health professional, you must usually respect the woman's decision, even if you feel it is the wrong one. In this situation, continue to educate the woman about PPD and options for its treatment, and follow up regularly in case she changes her mind or her symptoms worsen.

There are specific situations in which someone can undergo psychiatric care without his or her consent. All jurisdictions have mental health acts that allow a physician to mandate that someone undergo psychiatric observation and/or treatment. While the specific criteria vary from province to province, generally the requirement is that the person appears to be a danger to him- or herself or to others. However, mental health acts only govern the activities of physicians. For other service providers, most institutions/agencies will have protocols to follow in the case of someone who refuses care or appears to be at risk for suicide or homicide. You may also wish to check with your professional regulating body (e.g., College of Nurses) to find out how the Codes of Conduct or Standards of Practice that are relevant to you address this issue.

Finally, if a woman refuses a referral or treatment, you are *obligated* to notify child protection services if you are concerned that a child is or may be in need of protection.

ACCESSIBILITY OF SERVICES FOR WOMEN WITHOUT HEALTH INSURANCE

Provincial health insurance plans cover many health services for postpartum women, so most mothers will be able to access them free of charge. However, accessibility can be an issue for women who are **refugees**, have no legal status in Canada or do not otherwise have provincial health insurance.

You can help women who are eligible for health insurance to complete the required forms and procedures (see www.cic.gc.ca/english/newcomer/ fact_health.html#2). You could also make a list of community health care services that provide care to people without health insurance to give out to mothers. Discuss the woman's insurance status before making a referral to ensure that the services you suggest will be accessible to her.

ACCESSIBILITY OF SERVICES FOR WOMEN IN RURAL AND/OR REMOTE COMMUNITIES

In many rural and/or remote communities, people may have extremely limited access to mental health services. Many smaller communities have very infrequent access to specialized mental health service providers, such as psychiatrists or **psychologists**. In some places, it is even difficult to find a family physician.

In these communities, you may need to refer a woman with possible PPD to the nearest hospital emergency department or a walk-in clinic where a physician can assess her. You can then encourage the woman's treating physician to consult with experts in women's mental health care in larger communities to develop a treatment plan.

Many psychiatric services provide consultations to underserviced communities by videoconference or teleconference. In Ontario, you can contact the Ontario Psychiatric Outreach Program (see www.psychiatry.med.uwo.ca/ecp) to find out if this type of consultation is available in your area. Other parts of Canada have similar programs. Check with the medical school(s) nearest to you to find out whether or not this service is available.

What Role Do Various Services and Professionals Play in Assessing and Treating PPD?

The section that follows describes the role of various health care providers and services in the treatment and assessment of PPD.

HOSPITAL EMERGENCY DEPARTMENTS

What are they?

Hospital emergency departments provide assessment and initiate treatment for individuals with urgent concerns or in medical crisis. A triage nurse usually interviews patients. She or he determines the urgency of assessing each individual. An emergency room physician will then assess the patient, and call in specialists (e.g., psychiatrists, neurologists) if necessary and available. Patients may wait several hours to see an emergency room physician, and even longer to see a specialist.

What role can they play?

Hospital emergency departments play an important role in severe PPD and postpartum psychosis. As described above, the nearest hospital emergency department will be the usual source of referral in the case of suicidal ideation or possible psychotic symptoms. Hospital emergency staff will assess, admit if necessary or refer to a psychiatrist any women who present in the emergency department with these symptoms.

Hospital emergency staff probably won't admit a mother with mild to moderate PPD to a psychiatric unit for treatment; however, admission is much more likely for a woman with postpartum psychosis. A woman with severe PPD might be admitted to hospital if she also has a personality disorder or is refusing to take medication, or if there is a severe threat of harm to the woman or her baby. In the rare cases when a mother would need to be admitted, it is unlikely that the baby would accompany her. (Very few hospitals are equipped to house mothers and infants within the same unit.) In most cases, a mother with PPD who visits a hospital emergency room will receive a referral for care as an outpatient from a mental health professional.

How can a woman access emergency?
Anyone can walk into a hospital emergency department to receive medical
services. Provincial health insurance programs cover services provided, so there
is generally no cost to the person receiving care except for special services such
as ambulance transfer.

FAMILY PHYSICIANS AND GENERAL PRACTITIONERS

Who are they?
Family physicians and **general practitioners** are medical doctors who provide
preventive and general health care. Family physicians differ from general practitioners
in that they have completed special training in the field of family medicine. They are
not specialized in psychiatry, although some family doctors have obtained extra
training in psychotherapy. Some family doctors participate in "shared care" programs,
in which they work under the guidance of a psychiatrist to treat patients with mental
health concerns.

What role can they play?
Sometimes symptoms are not severe enough to warrant emergency referral, but a
patient requires further assessment. In such cases, a service provider should refer the
patient to a family doctor. If the woman has an established relationship with a family
doctor, that doctor will generally be familiar with what the woman is usually like, and
so will be able to recognize changes from her usual personality. The family doctor also
plays an important role in ruling out other potential problems that could be causing
the symptoms of depression (e.g., thyroid dysfunction) by ordering the necessary tests.

Most family physicians and general practitioners are trained to diagnose
depression, and many will provide treatment (usually antidepressants). However,
instead of themselves providing treatment, some family doctors will make a
referral to a psychiatrist, or may request that a psychiatrist assess the woman;
the psychiatrist will then offer the family doctor recommendations about what
treatment to prescribe. This is particularly common if the woman does not respond
to treatment initiated by the family physician or if the woman is breastfeeding her
infant and is concerned about potential effects of antidepressants.

How can a woman access a family doctor?

If the woman has a family doctor, you can encourage her to phone herself to make an appointment with her physician, or you can phone the family doctor directly (you should seek the woman's permission before doing this—find out about the agency's informed consent policy).

For women who do not have a family doctor, a doctor in a walk-in clinic or emergency room can also rule out physical causes of the symptoms, and make a psychiatric referral if necessary. To help find someone a family doctor in Ontario, you can call the Find a Doctor service through the College of Physicians and Surgeons of Ontario: 416 967-2626 in Toronto or toll-free at 1 800 268-7096. Or you can view their website at www.cpso.on.ca/Doctor_Search/dr_srch_hm.htm. For outside of Ontario, the website www.physician.info/MD_CD.HTM provides a link to the appropriate province or territory.

The provincial health insurance programs cover services provided to residents of Canada by family doctors.

PSYCHIATRISTS

Who are they?

Psychiatrists are medical doctors who also have at least five years of specialized training in mental health. Some psychiatrists work in independent practices, and others are affiliated with hospital departments of psychiatry. Some psychiatrists work specifically with PPD or women's mental health more generally. Other psychiatrists are particularly experienced in prescribing psychiatric medications or providing various types of psychotherapy. People may wait two months or more to see a psychiatrist, although psychiatrists usually prioritize new clients and may be able to see a woman who has recently had a baby earlier.

What role can they play?

For women with severe PPD, psychiatrists will usually be the primary treatment providers. They will first complete a thorough review of the woman's medical and mental health history and then find out about her current symptoms to make a formal diagnosis of PPD. If needed, they will also order tests to rule out any other contributors to her symptoms. Then, together with the woman, her family, and sometimes her family doctor or general practitioner, the psychiatrist will recommend treatment. Psychiatric treatment will usually involve taking antidepressants (or other medications), getting psychotherapy or a combination of both, though some psychiatrists may recommend other treatment options as described in Chapter 5.

How can a woman be seen by a psychiatrist?

Women usually need to be referred by a family doctor or general practitioner, although psychiatrists affiliated with some mental health clinics will accept a self-referral or referral from health care providers who are not physicians. As described above, a walk-in clinic or hospital emergency department can also give a woman a psychiatric referral if she has no family doctor.

Some communities may not have psychiatrists. In this case, refer the woman to the nearest major centre, or she may have to wait to see a visiting psychiatrist. Some communities have implemented video assessment services in order to complete psychiatric assessments without requiring travel. To help find someone a psychiatrist in Ontario, you can call the College of Physicians and Surgeons of Ontario at 416 967-2626 in Toronto or toll-free at 1 800 268-7096. Or you can view their website at www.cpso.on.ca/Doctor_Search/dr_srch_hm.htm.

Psychiatrists generally bill provincial health plans for their services, so there is usually no cost.

PSYCHOLOGISTS

Who are they?

Clinical psychologists have at least nine years of university education, and at least one year of supervised clinical practice. They are trained in making diagnoses and providing psychotherapy. They are not licensed to prescribe medication. Like psychiatrists, they may work in a private practice, or they may be affiliated with a hospital, community agency, school or workplace. Also like psychiatrists, they are regulated by a provincial governing body (in Ontario, the College of Psychologists of Ontario).

What role can they play?

For women with PPD who choose to be treated with psychotherapy, a psychologist may be the primary treatment provider.

How can a woman be seen by a psychologist?

Most psychologists allow for self-referral. However, unless psychologists are affiliated with a medical clinic, provincial health insurance programs do not cover their services, which may result in a substantial cost to the patient if she does not have a private insurance plan. The Ontario Psychological Association at 416 961-0069 in Toronto or toll-free at 1 800 268-0069 has information about how to find a psychologist in Ontario. The Canadian Psychological Association website www.cpa.ca has information about how to find a psychologist outside of Ontario.

OTHER MENTAL HEALTH SERVICE PROVIDERS

Who are they?

Other service providers, including social workers, nurses and occupational therapists, may offer mental health counselling independently, or may work as part of a mental health clinic, employee assistance program or school counselling office. The training of these providers varies depending on their field of specialty, and can range from a diploma to a PhD. Besides these health professionals, there are also non-licensed "psychotherapists," who offer mental health care in private practices. However, it is important to note that since these therapists are not licensed, no regulations govern their training or quality of care.

What role can they play?

These service providers may have the training to offer psychotherapy, or they may work together with a psychiatrist to offer a more holistic treatment plan for a woman with PPD.

How can a woman be seen by other mental health providers?

The woman's family doctor, general practitioner or psychiatrist may recommend mental health service providers, or these providers may work as part of the mental health clinic where the woman is receiving treatment. The Canadian Association of Social Workers website at www.casw-acts.ca offers information about how to find a social worker.

PUBLIC HEALTH NURSES

Who are they?

Public health nurses are registered nurses whose practice promotes the health of individuals, families, communities and populations. Public health nurses have an undergraduate degree in nursing and are regulated by provincial agencies. Cities, regions or provinces can employ public health nurses. Some public health nurses have a generalist practice and others may work exclusively with families with young children, including expectant families. Education and training related to mental health issues, including PPD, vary widely depending on the setting and the individual nurse's needs and interests.

What role can they play?

The role that public health nurses play in detection, prevention and treatment of PPD varies depending on the local public health mandate, as well as the resources available within both the public health unit and the community at large. Public health may offer a range of PPD-related services, sometimes in collaboration with other health or community-based agencies. These services may include screening (either targeted or universal, as discussed in Chapter 3), assessment, referral to mental health and other services, advocacy, service co-ordination, support and psychoeducational groups and provision of home visiting programs, which may include support and/or counselling.

How can a woman be seen by a public health nurse?

Contact information for each local public health office appears in the local telephone book and/or on the Internet. In most cases, women can self-refer for public health services, and programs/services are available free of charge.

PPD SUPPORT GROUPS

What are they?

PPD support groups may be of two types: those organized and facilitated by women who are not mental health professionals but who have experienced PPD, or those organized and facilitated by professionals, usually in affiliation with a hospital, health clinic, not-for-profit organization or public health unit. Support groups usually meet weekly and may be open (i.e., women are free to attend as many or as few weeks of the group as they like) or closed (i.e., the group will run for a fixed number of weeks, usually with a different topic planned for each session, and women are asked to commit to attending all or most group meetings).

What role can they play?

PPD support groups provide the important function of giving women with PPD a comfortable and supportive place to discuss their feelings and experiences. They also give women a chance to develop support networks of mothers with young children. Women with mild PPD may not require any intervention other than attending a support group. For women with moderate or severe PPD, support groups are often an important complement to the individual medical or psychological treatment they receive.

How can a woman access a support group?

Listings of PPD support groups appear on the website for Our Sister's Place (www.oursistersplace.ca/info/PDF/ppdsupportgroups.pdf) or at www.postpartum.org/supportgroups.html. Some public health units and community health centres offer PPD support groups; contact information for local agencies can be found in the telephone book. Most support groups encourage the mother to self-refer, although there may be a waiting list. Most groups run out of hospitals, public health units or community health centres are free of charge. Some support groups may charge a fee.

MENTAL HEALTH CRISIS AND OTHER TELEPHONE LINES

What are they?

Counsellors (usually trained volunteers) staff distress or crisis telephone lines 24 hours daily. They offer free, anonymous telephone counselling and referral for individuals in a mental health crisis. Nurses staff other 24-hour health information lines (e.g., Telehealth Ontario, Info-santé in Québec) and can offer emergency telephone counselling and referral.

What role can they play?

It is a good idea to include a list of mental health crisis lines as part of a resource list for any mothers with PPD or suspected PPD. Service providers should encourage mothers to phone a crisis line if ever they feel overwhelmed and they do not have access to their usual medical or social supports. Crisis lines provide a useful backup plan, but will not substitute for a referral to and treatment by a mental health professional.

How can a woman speak with a counsellor?

A list of crisis lines appears in Appendix D (page 157).

Summary

A woman should receive a referral for PPD treatment or assessment whenever she herself, her family members or her service providers feel that she may be depressed. More specific guidelines for referral appear in Figure 6–1. *The service provider must ensure that a woman who is having persistent suicidal thoughts or symptoms of psychosis follows through on the referral for an emergency psychiatric assessment. She should not be left by herself or alone with the baby until this assessment occurs.* (See page 62 on emergency referrals.)

A woman with PPD can be referred to a psychiatrist, a family doctor or general practitioner, or any of the other health care providers and services listed on pages 70 to 76, depending on availability in each community and the nature and severity of her symptoms. (See Figure 6–1.)

7
Impact on the Family

How does postpartum depression affect the father or partner?

How can the partner or family help a mother with postpartum depression?

Can new fathers or partners develop depression?

How might a mother's depression affect her infant?

Pregnancy and childbirth typically entail vast emotional and physical upheaval, not only for the child-bearing mother but also for her family and those close to her. In traditional families, the person closest to the mother is usually the baby's father. However, in today's Western society, families are diverse: mothers may not have a partner, the mother's partner may not be the infant's biological father, the mother may have a **lesbian** partner, and extended family members or people who are not biological kin may be considered important parts of the family unit.

The changes and stresses associated with a new baby can take a toll not only on the mental health of the mother but also on her partner or other close family members. In addition, some research has reported an association between **postpartum depression (PPD)** and problems in **cognitive** and social development of the infant.

This chapter reviews the impact of PPD on partners, infants and other family members.

Severe PPD Affects All Family Members

For the people close to a mother with severe PPD, living with and witnessing her hopelessness and dejected mood can be an intense emotional experience. Her partner and other family members may question their own role in her illness. They may feel insecure, uncertain how to manage the problem, powerless to help and fearful for the mother's and baby's safety. Some describe it like "walking on eggshells" or "never being sure what will happen next."

Dealing with a person who is depressed can be very taxing; one must call on deep inner resources to cope with the situation. The partner and relatives of a mother with PPD may feel constantly worried yet also exasperated, finding their patience worn thin in handling the situation. For the partner and relatives, trying to carry on with their own lives while comforting and supporting the mother with depression is no easy matter.

Partners and Family Members Need Information about PPD

Many partners might never have heard of PPD and so will need information about its prevalence, symptoms and the fact that it requires treatment as well as ways in which they might help in detecting the condition should it occur. A partner's or family member's careful eye might help ensure that a mother with PPD receives treatment promptly.

Like mothers themselves, partners and family members may have bought into the myth that mothers will be happy all the time. Because of this, they may become concerned about even normal fluctuations in the mother's mood. On the other hand, they may dismiss symptoms of depression as the "blues," and in doing so, discourage the mother from seeking treatment when she needs it. Partners often have unrealistic expectations about what looking after an infant entails, and may unwittingly contribute to a mother's distress by criticizing her appearance or an untidy house. While marital conflict or relationship problems during pregnancy and in the perinatal period are risk factors for the development of PPD (see Chapter 2), the reverse is also true. Parenting a baby can also strain the relationship, as being parents alters the family's lifestyle, compelling partners to take on additional responsibilities and adopt new roles.

Partners or family members can receive information about PPD either directly or through the mother's service providers. Numerous PPD resources for partners are also available on the Internet (see, for example, www.postpartum.net/fathers.html). Once partners or family members know that PPD may occur, the mother's partner (and close family members) can watch for warning signs of depression, such as anxiety, low mood and a loss of pleasure in things usually enjoyed (see Chapter 1); the mother can then begin treatment immediately if these symptoms develop.

Fathers, partners or other family members can provide valuable information to health care professionals, alerting them and giving them clues to the possibility of PPD, especially when the mother herself is reluctant to divulge the extent of her despair. The woman's partner and close family members are in a unique position to observe the mother's depressed state and make her aware that she may need professional attention.

Partner Support Is Invaluable

Research suggests that a partner's support may help to protect the mother from PPD (Eberhard-Gran et al., 2002). Both during pregnancy and after the birth, a partner's support can decrease the mother's chances of developing PPD or lessen its severity and accelerate her recovery. Some research suggests that the greater the partner's involvement in the mother's treatment, the quicker her recovery is likely to be (Misri et al., 2000). Although no research has specifically evaluated the effects of support from family members other than the partner, important benefits are likely to result from this type of support as well (Eberhard-Gran et al., 2002).

By understanding why the mother and her service provider have selected a certain treatment and by sharing in the therapy, the partner and family members can endorse the mother's chosen method of dealing with her depression. Also important is that the partner and family members be non-judgmental listeners: many women who are depressed feel that they have no one to talk to who will understand them. Partners and family members can let the woman know that they will support her through this, that they are there for her and that they love her. An open-minded, sympathetic attitude is best, with the partner and family members reassuring the mother that she is doing her best and that she will recover.

If the partner and other family members can take on as many of the baby care and household jobs as possible, the mother then has an opportunity to rest. They can also organize help from others (relatives, friends or community respite care programs) for baby care, housework, shopping, meal preparation and looking after older siblings. If family members or friends can help, the mother and her partner may also find it therapeutic to have some "couple time" without the baby.

SUGGESTIONS FOR THE PARTNER AND FAMILY TO HELP MOTHERS WITH PPD

As a partner or family member, what you can say or do to help the mother overwhelmed by PPD:

- Help her to work with her doctor or other health care providers to make informed decisions about which treatment plan is the best one for her.
- Inquire what works best for her and which kind of support she prefers; ask for "a script" or list delineating how people can help the most.
- Help out with tasks without waiting to be asked (she will always appreciate your washing dishes, doing laundry or preparing meals).
- Assure her that you will get through it together, that you're there for her, that you know she's doing her best and that you love her.
- Encourage her to talk openly about her feelings; show her that you understand or are doing your best to understand.
- Tell her that the depression is not her fault, she's not to blame—it is *not* within her control.

As a partner or family member, what is best not to do or say:

- Don't comment on an unclean house, unwashed clothes or other things she has left undone. *(It only exacerbates her own sense of guilt and worthlessness.)*
- Don't avoid spending time with her, even when it seems difficult or uncomfortable. *(She likely feels very alone and appreciates you being near by.)*
- Avoid criticizing her housekeeping or how she looks after the baby. *(She may already worry about being an unworthy or useless mother.)*
- Don't compare her with other family members and friends. *(Everyone's experience with a new baby is different.)*
- Don't say:
  - "Think about the things you have to be happy about." *(She knows that!)*
  - "Snap out of it." *(She would if she could; no one would want to feel the way she does.)*
- [For the partner or spouse] Don't criticize her appearance; try to be physically affectionate and reassuring, without asking for sex. *(She's likely feeling unattractive.)*

Fathers' and/or Partners' Reactions to Parenthood and PPD

All new parents are likely to have many worries and concerns prior to and following the birth of a baby (Gage & Kirk, 2002). Fathers and/or partners may feel an increased sense of responsibility; they may wonder whether or not the baby's arrival will create havoc in their lives and how it will affect their sexual relationship with the mother. They may worry about their abilities to provide financially for the new member of the family, their proficiency in caring for a baby, the curtailment of their free time, and their disrupted sleep. Some partners also have ambivalent feelings about breastfeeding.

Even when fathers and/or partners fully intend to take on a fair share of the parenting duties, they can find it difficult to do so, particularly when the mother is breastfeeding. They usually end up doing far less of the child care and household chores than the mother. Consequently, mothers commonly feel that their partners are not "pulling their weight," or that their partners take the mothering job for granted. Often, both partners have trouble knowing and expressing what they need at this time, further straining the relationship.

Partners may experience role confusion, feel ignored, rejected and excluded from the close mother-baby relationship. They may feel that the mother "shuts them out" of the baby's life, and that health care professionals do not actively include them in decision-making about the birth and child care.

Partners of mothers with PPD often fear the relationship will never again be "like it was." Upset by the mother with depression, many partners feel useless because they cannot alleviate her suffering. Some report a sense of powerlessness and frustration at being unable to "fix" the problem, not realizing there is no quick-fix remedy.

Service providers can help partners to realize that:
• they should not take the mother's illness personally
• it is not their fault that the mother is depressed
• they did not cause the mother's PPD
• they cannot remove or cure the PPD, which requires professional treatment
• they can help by listening, offering support and organizing help from others
• they too need a break.

Service providers can provide guidance, emphasizing the partner's valuable contribution to both the mother's and baby's well-being. Some centres offer groups for partners of women with PPD, to give them a forum to discuss their concerns with others who are facing similar issues. Caregivers can educate partners and/or fathers about the crucial role their support plays in helping the mother overcome her depression. Service providers must maintain patient confidentiality when discussing a woman's situation with her family, and seek the mother's permission before sharing any details about her condition. However, even without sharing any sensitive information, service providers can reinforce and bolster partners and/or fathers in their efforts to support a mother who is severely depressed, because doing so can be very exhausting work.

Postpartum Distress in Fathers and/or Partners

Researchers and health care providers have debated whether or not it is appropriate to apply the term "postpartum depression," or PPD, to a parent who has not given birth to a child. Those who believe that the hormonal changes accompanying the postpartum period are the primary explanation for PPD argue that it cannot be said to develop in non–child-bearing parents, including fathers. Others, however, note that the father or co-parent experiences many of the stresses experienced by a woman in the post-birth period (e.g., role changes, sleep disruption), perhaps leaving the father or co-parent vulnerable to depression as well. To address this question, some researchers have explored the mental health of fathers during the postpartum period, and a review of this research follows.

A recent review (Goodman, 2004) identified 20 studies of "paternal depression" (depression in fathers) during the first year postpartum. Depending upon how researchers measured depression, they classified approximately 12 to 13 per cent of fathers in community samples as depressed. In assessing partners of women diagnosed with PPD, researchers found that as many as one-quarter had depression or other psychiatric problems (Zelkowitz & Milet, 2001).

Many studies have identified PPD in the mother as the strongest predictor of depression in fathers of new babies (Matthey et al., 2000; Areias et al., 1996). Other predictors of paternal depression include a personal history of depression, the quality of the couple's relationship and socio-economic status (reviewed in Goodman, 2004).

Some research has suggested that depression in fathers with new babies may follow a different course than in mothers; at least one study suggests that the onset is usually later, and the rate increases over the first postpartum year. Paternal depression can be long-lasting: of fathers who are depressed at six to eight weeks postpartum, 50 to 60 per cent remain depressed at six months postpartum (Matthey et al., 2000).

Researchers have not developed any screening tools specifically to measure depression in men following the birth of a baby. They have used the **Edinburgh Postnatal Depression Scale (EPDS)** in most studies of paternal depression, but there is evidence that men respond differently to this tool than women do (Matthey et al., 2001). In a study of 208 fathers and 230 mothers, fathers endorsed seven of the 10 items on the EPDS less frequently than did mothers, with the most striking difference being on the EPDS item "so unhappy I have been crying." (Fathers were much less likely to respond positively to this item.)

These differences in the symptoms reported by men and women in the post-partum period are similar to differences in symptoms of depression seen between men and women in general. They likely result from the different socially accepted ways that men and women express distress; while depression and tearfulness are common in women, men may be more likely to exhibit their distress as anxiety, substance abuse or aggression.

Researchers still have to identify the reasons for the high rates of depression in partners of women with PPD. Possibly both partners become depressed in response to shared family variables (e.g., a difficult or ill infant, relationship dissatisfaction) or shared variables unrelated to the family (e.g., socio-economic status), or perhaps people who are vulnerable to depression are more likely to engage in a relationship together. However, it is also possible that fathers whose partners have PPD develop depression or anxiety in response to the worry and stress associated with taking on the primary responsibility for the care of both their partners and their infants.

Possible Impact of PPD on the Infant

Women with PPD are understandably concerned about the possible effects of depression on their babies, particularly as many women already feel anxious about being bad mothers.

Studies indicate that prolonged, or chronic, untreated PPD *may* hamper mother-infant attachment, and could possibly hinder the child's cognitive and behavioural development (particularly language skills and IQ), more so in boys than girls (Sharp et al., 1995; Murray et al., 1996; Murray & Cooper, 1997).

However, exposure to chronic and long-lasting, or recurrent and severe, maternal depression seems to affect infant development, rather than just one postpartum episode (Murray & Cooper, 1997). In addition, methodological problems make it difficult to confirm that the differences noted in children of mothers who had PPD actually resulted from the mothers' depression, rather than from other variables (e.g., genetic risk for depression, other psychiatric problems in both the mother and child, or **stressors** such as poverty, unsafe or unstable housing, marital conflict, domestic violence or abuse).

Moreover, how a mother's PPD affects her infant will vary according to many factors: the duration of her illness, the baby's temperament, and how much others, such as the baby's father (or the mother's partner or parents), provide affection and participate in child care. Strong attachment between the partner and the infant can help to promote the child's optimal development.

When working with mothers who are depressed, service providers need to remember that any discussion of possible negative outcomes for the baby or an overemphasis on attachment will only exacerbate the mothers' feelings of despondency, guilt and inadequacy. It is important to educate mothers that PPD, in and of itself, probably does not "cause" problems in children. Rather, PPD can (but doesn't always) impair a mother's ability to interact with her infant in healthy and consistent ways. Infant massage or specialized mother-baby programs for women with PPD may help mothers with depression to interact more confidently with their babies.

Impact of PPD on Other Family Members

No research studies have specifically evaluated the impact of PPD on other family members, such as older children in the family, the mother's parents or other extended family members. However, research indicates that depression in general can have significant and diverse effects on family members and caregivers.

Changes in their mothers' mood and behaviour could affect older children of mothers with PPD. Studies of toddlers, school-aged children and adolescents have provided some evidence that children of mothers who are depressed show more negative outcomes, including behaviour problems and psychiatric diagnoses, compared with children whose mothers are not depressed (Cicchetti et al., 1998; Hammen & Brennan, 2003). The effects of PPD on newborn infants are likely influenced by many variables, including genetic risk for depression and other psychopathology; characteristics of the child, such as temperament; and the quality of the social environment (Goodman & Gotlib, 1999).

Researchers who have studied the effects of maternal depression on children emphasize the importance of acknowledging that many children of mothers who are depressed seem to be resilient to negative outcomes (Brennan et al., 2003). Involvement of a father or another caregiver may foster this resilience (Goodman & Gotlib, 1999).

All those who care for a woman with PPD, including grandparents and other family members, need to be mindful of the toll their caregiving responsibilities may be taking on their own mental health. The demands of caring for the mother, and perhaps her baby as well, are bound, at times, to be associated with feelings of stress and exhaustion. Service providers should encourage all caregivers to take breaks, to try to maintain their own pleasurable activities as much as is feasible and, if necessary, to seek support for their own frustrations and concerns. Support groups for caregivers of people with depression are available in many areas. (See Appendix D at the end of this guide.)

Summary

As with depression that occurs at any other time in life, PPD can significantly strain relationships. Educating and keeping the partner involved in the mother's treatment may help to hasten her recovery and strengthen the couple's ties.

Partners and other family members can help a mother with PPD by taking on as much of the household work and baby care as possible, by being good listeners, and by reassuring her that they love her and she will recover.

The early weeks and months with a new baby are stressful for all parents, and particularly if the mother has PPD. Partners need to look after their own mental health as well, and should consult health care providers if they notice symptoms of depression or anxiety.

Although a mother's PPD *might* undermine her child's cognitive, social and behavioural development, the impairment stems from chronic depression, not from a single time-limited episode of PPD.

8
Issues for Specific Populations of Postpartum Women

What populations may have unique mental health needs during the postpartum period?

What strategies can service providers use to ensure that they meet the needs of all women who require PPD-related services?

Most of the research on the identification, prevention and treatment of **postpartum depression (PPD)** has relied predominantly on samples of heterosexual Caucasian women in stable relationships, living in urban communities in Western nations. However, these groups form only a small proportion of the women having babies in many health care settings.

This chapter provides a summary of the research and some clinical suggestions for working with women whose specific needs may not be met by traditional programs for PPD assessment and treatment.

These groups include:
• women of diverse ethnocultural origins, and particularly **immigrant** and **refugee** women
• women from rural or remote communities
• women who use alcohol and other substances
• women who have experienced physical or sexual abuse
• **Aboriginal** women
• adolescent and single mothers

- **lesbian** mothers
- adoptive mothers
- women with chronic mental illnesses or other disabilities.

Unless specifically noted, discussion of these particular populations in this chapter should not imply that these women are at any greater or lesser risk of PPD than other women. Rather, we wish to highlight that service providers should be aware that these women may have unique needs related to PPD assessment and referral.

Women of Diverse Ethnocultural Origins

Canada is home to women of diverse ethnic origins, and different cultures have different beliefs and traditions, not only about childbirth, but also regarding mental illness. For these reasons, service providers need to consider other unique factors when working with women with depression who come from culturally diverse populations.

Recent research suggests that women from non-Western cultures experience postpartum mood problems at approximately the same rates as those in Western countries (O'Hara, 1994). However, some studies find higher rates of PPD among immigrant groups than in native-born populations (see below). Research to date indicates that risk factors for PPD are generally consistent across different ethno-cultural groups. Among the risk factors for PPD, prenatal depression and lack of social support are consistently most prominent in many ethnocultural groups. For instance, this is true of Lebanese women in Beirut (Chaaya et al., 2002), Mexican-American women in the United States (Martinez-Schallmoser et al., 2003) and Indian women in Goa (Patel et al., 2002).

Researchers have also reported some culturally-specific risk factors for PPD. In particular, they have linked infant sex to increased risks of PPD among women in India and Hong Kong (Rodrigues et al., 2003; Patel et al., 2002), mainly owing to the women's preference for male offspring. One Indian study found that women who expressed a preference for giving birth to a boy were at increased risk for other adverse outcomes, including marital violence, likely because of pressure from their husbands or in-laws (Patel et al., 2002).

Other culturally-specific family variables that have been identified as possible risk factors include lack of instrumental support from the baby's father, based on research in India (Rodrigues et al., 2003), and a poor relationship with in-laws, based on research in Turkey (Danaci et al., 2002). However, one could argue that these variables are equally relevant and exacerbating factors for PPD in Western cultures, considering the strong link between a lack of social or partner support and PPD. Researchers need to do more work to better understand risk factors for PPD in diverse ethnocultural groups.

Motherhood in Immigrant and Refugee Populations

An *immigrant* is a person who leaves her/his native country to settle in another country. Mothers of new babies who are also recent immigrants to a host country face significant psychosocial stresses that service providers must take into account when assessing and treating PPD. In a multifactorial predictive study completed by Dennis, recently arrived immigrant women were five times more likely to develop depressive symptoms in the early postpartum period than were mothers who were born in Canada (Dennis et al., 2004).

In adapting to their host country, immigrant women face many challenges, such as learning a new language, adapting to unfamiliar customs, adjusting to a different manner of social interaction, and accepting new rules and laws. Immigrant women who give birth in their new country may face a clash between the Western "myth of motherhood" (in which the mother supposedly cares competently for herself and her new infant, essentially without help) and the view of motherhood in the home culture, which would often involve more social and/or family assistance (Barclay & Kent, 1998).

A *refugee* is a person who has left his or her country of origin out of fear of being persecuted on the basis of race, religion, political opinion or another characteristic of her or his identity. Although refugee women share many of the same concerns as non-refugee immigrants (e.g., isolation from family, language barriers), refugee women also have some unique issues that may be relevant to their mental health during the postpartum period. Specifically, refugee women may have been victims of torture or sex- and gender-based violence, including rape. Their arrival in the host country is often unplanned and involuntary, and many will have left loved ones behind. Most refugees do not have the option of returning to their countries of origin (Gagnon et al., 2004). These additional issues may well contribute to distress in the postpartum period.

Presentation of Depressive Symptoms in Diverse Ethnocultural Groups

The presentation, or symptom profile, of depression can vary in different cultures. It is widely held that some groups may express more physical, or somatic, versus emotional, or affective, symptoms of depression. **Somatization** has been reported to be a common way to express depression among Asian and African cultures, while complaints of sadness, together with guilt, are more characteristic of depression in Western cultures. This difference could lead to difficulties in screening for and diagnosing depression in non-Western populations if Western-developed tools are being used.

However, recent international research has found no consistent geographic differences in somatization of depression. In fact, researchers found that variables other than ethnicity and culture, including whether or not an individual had a consistent relationship with a health care provider, were better predictors of which depressive symptoms an individual reported (Simon et al., 1999). One recent study of PPD in Vietnamese, Turkish and Filipino women living in Australia found no consistent differences in rates of somatization between these immigrant populations and Australian-born women (Small et al., 2003). Therefore, service providers should not make assumptions about which symptoms to anticipate in dealing with specific ethnocultural groups.

The **Edinburgh Postnatal Depression Scale (EPDS)** and **Postpartum Depression Screening Scale (PDSS)** are tools used to detect PPD. Although they are translated into various languages, may give different and sometimes unreliable results when in forms other than the original English-language version. This can occur because of the tools' use of words or phrases that cannot be literally translated in some languages (e.g., in the EPDS, "things have been getting on top of me"). Since the questions may carry slightly different meanings in translation, and as a result of potential cross-cultural differences in expression of depressive symptoms, appropriate cut-off scores may vary for different populations (see Cox & Holden, 2003). Finally, researchers and clinicians working in cross-cultural psychiatry debate the degree to which the concept of PPD, or even depression, has meaning within certain ethnocultural groups. Those using screening tools to assess populations other than English-speaking Caucasian women—for whom most screening tools have been developed—must interpret scores in the appropriate cultural context, and also rely on other assessment procedures, including clinical judgment (see also Chapter 3).

How Childbirth Rituals May Protect Women from PPD in Some Cultural Groups

In many cultures, childbirth is accompanied by a series of rituals or traditions intended to safeguard the health of the mother and her baby. Quite often, these traditions involve a period of rest and seclusion for the mother in the weeks or months following childbirth, with female relatives and neighbours looking after the mother and newborn. One example is the Chinese custom of "doing the month," which is a period of rest, seclusion and dietary restriction, while a female relative (usually the mother-in-law) helps care for the woman and her family (Steinberg, 1996).

Some researchers have speculated that such traditions, which effectively shield the mother from the physical and emotional burden of baby care during the early postpartum weeks, may protect her from PPD. By imposing structure and meaning in the perinatal period, such traditions may facilitate the transition to parenthood. However, some women may find the seclusion associated with these rituals to be isolating and an indicator of their lack of personal control over their own and their babies' lives; researchers need to further investigate this possibility. From either perspective, service providers need to consider these practices as potential determinants of postpartum mental health (Stern & Kruckman, 1983).

Participating in childbirth rituals or traditions may also have implications for the detection and treatment of PPD. Based on their research with women in China, Lee and colleagues have speculated that "doing the month" may simply postpone the onset of significant depressive symptoms beyond six weeks postpartum (i.e., until after the mother resumes her caretaking responsibilities) (Lee et al., 1998).

Researchers have examined these postpartum rituals in varying degrees among indigenous Arabic (Hundt et al., 2000; Nahas & Amasheh, 1999), Chinese (Holroyd et al., 1997; Lee et al., 1998), Japanese (Yoshida et al., 2001), Malaysian (Kit et al., 1997), Taiwanese (Huang & Mathers, 2001) and Thai (Kaewsarn et al., 2003) women. The postpartum rituals often last 30 to 40 days: they include organized support, stringent dietary measures, hygiene practices (to preserve the health of mother and baby) and restricted physical activities (Hundt et al., 2000; Matthey et al., 2002).

A study of Jewish women living in Jerusalem found a decreasing trend for PPD among the more traditional, religious and orthodox sections of that society. The authors of this study suggest that PPD symptoms may develop less frequently, or are easier to cope with, in religious women because of the more cohesive social structure, emphasis on rituals and greater community support (Dankner et al., 2000).

In immigrant populations, however, childbirth traditions can also be a source of stress. This is particularly true if the woman does not have enough support or resources to adhere to or participate in practices that she believes are important to her own or her baby's health. If a woman cannot, or decides not to, participate in her cultural traditions, she may attribute future symptoms of depression to her failure to do so, or she may experience disapproval from members of her cultural community.

Access to and Use of Health Services among Immigrants

Canadian research has shown that immigrants are less likely than native-born Canadians to use specialized mental health services (Hyman, 2001). Immigrants often turn instead to primary caregivers or to informal sources, such as clergy, traditional healers, family and friends (Gallo et al., 1995; Peifer et al., 2000). This may occur because the Canadian health care system often does not accommodate non-Western beliefs about the significance and treatment of mental illness: immigrants may find or expect that Canadian health care providers will not understand their culture and therefore will not be able to help them.

Some individuals and communities will take up new beliefs or practices sooner than others, depending on the degree to which they are acculturated. They will likely fall somewhere along the continuum of understanding symptoms of mental illness according to what is typical in their home culture and according to what is typical in their new culture. Immigrants, refugees and other members of minority populations may face significant barriers in accessing appropriate mental health care, including language barriers, lack of information about available services, cultural insensitivity on the part of service providers, and financial obstacles. As a result of these barriers, women may be very reluctant to disclose their symptoms of depression.

STRATEGIES FOR WORKING WITH IMMIGRANT AND REFUGEE WOMEN

- Seek out diversity and/or cultural communications/sensitivity training to enhance your ability to provide culturally appropriate care to postpartum women. These courses will provide you with strategies for communicating with immigrant and refugee women to determine how best to meet their needs in the context of their cultural heritage. Many health units and hospitals offer diversity training and there are also some good resources online.
- Help a new immigrant to establish connections with other members of her home culture living in the host country. Many large immigrant communities run programs specifically for immigrant families with children.
- Reach out to diverse communities by working in partnership with community-based agencies. Partners within the communities of interest can help you to determine the types of programs needed (both in terms of services to mothers and education for the community) and how best to disseminate material.
- Disseminate information about the Canadian health care system, particularly as it relates to maternity and infant care (labour and delivery practices, vaccinations, etc.). You can provide this information either in print form or through a translator in the language that the woman understands best.

- Make information about PPD and support services available in as many languages as possible. Develop education campaigns in partnership with community agencies, and make use of local ethnic media. If your program does not have or is not able to develop these resources, other programs may be willing to share resources already developed.

PPD among Women in Rural and Remote Communities

Women living in rural, and particularly remote communities will generally be less likely to have easy access to nearby health care and social services. Because of barriers these women face in accessing health care, they may experience delays in getting appropriate PPD treatment, so that depressive symptoms are more severe by the time the women actually receive professional care (Lane et al., 2001).

Health professionals know little about the prevalence, risk factors or treatment of PPD in rural areas in Canada, as all the existing research comes from Australia and New Zealand. Prevalence rates reported are contradictory, and include rates that are higher (Griepsma et al., 1994; Johnstone et al., 2001), lower (Astbury et al., 1994) and no different from rates for women living in urban areas (Romans-Clarkson et al., 1990).

Service providers often assume that women living in rural communities are more socially isolated than women living in cities. However, while they may be geographically isolated, people in rural communities may be more likely than their urban counterparts to have immediate family close by and to be willing to use family and friends for help and support (Amato, 1993). Women living in remote communities, however, will be less likely to have family and friends nearby to provide support. Where social isolation is a problem, face-to-face social networks could be substituted by telephone support from a trained peer volunteer (Dennis, 2003a) or Internet chat rooms (e.g., www.ppdsupportpage.com) for women who have access to telephone and/or the Internet. Not all Internet chat rooms have moderators, so service providers should investigate their quality before recommending them.

The only study on treating PPD in a rural community found that a 10-week group therapy program, with a strong cognitive-behavioural component, was effective in a small sample of women (Lane et al., 2001). The study's authors point out that educating the community, including its health professionals, is an essential first step in promoting appropriate referral and PPD treatment. They also suggest that women in rural communities may believe some of the prevailing myths about motherhood—particularly the myth that mothering comes naturally or instinctively—even more strongly than their urban counterparts. Therefore, service providers may need to do more work in providing women with realistic ideas about parenting.

There may also be other barriers to women accessing treatment for PPD in rural areas. For instance, boundaries between professionals and their clients or patients may be more difficult to uphold in tightly knit rural communities, and mothers may be reluctant to participate in a group that likely includes women they know or meet regularly. As well, the community may be so small that there are not enough mothers with PPD at any one time to offer a support group.

STRATEGIES FOR WORKING WITH RURAL AND REMOTE POPULATIONS

• Offer PPD support through methods other than face-to-face. Many programs use telephone support, though you should take care to develop an "emergency plan" upon the initial contact. The plan might include an agreement to go to the nearest hospital emergency department if she or the service provider feels it is necessary and a list of family members, health care providers or crisis lines the woman can call in an emergency situation if she cannot reach her usual telephone support person. This kind of plan will prove useful should the woman at some point require urgent face-to-face care.

• Suggest Internet support (e.g., through Our Sisters' Place). This is a new development and may prove very useful to women with Internet access. (See p. 158 for more information on Our Sisters' Place.)

• Develop clear boundaries upon the first contact (e.g., Is it appropriate for the woman to call or visit you at home? Should you address one another if you meet in public and, if so, how should you do so?). These boundaries may differ from usual boundaries in an urban centre, where providers are much less likely to meet clients or patients outside of the medical/therapeutic setting.

• Recognize that PPD support groups may be more difficult to establish in rural communities, since women know that they are likely to be in the same group with friends or acquaintances. When founders establish groups, they need to outline clear rules of confidentiality (as above). They may also choose to have the rules of confidentiality available in written form to reassure a woman who is nervous about attending the group.

• Consider alternatives for communities too small to sustain a support group. In those communities, one-on-one support by trained peer volunteers or service providers (either face to face or via telephone) may be an option.

PPD in Women Who Use Substances

Major depression rates are high among women accessing treatment for substance use, perhaps due to high rates of current or past physical or sexual abuse or low socio-economic status.

Depression may be a precursor to, or a consequence of, substance use. For example, women with significant symptoms of depression may self-medicate with alcohol or illicit drugs. Depression-like symptoms can also arise from using substances such as alcohol, which can cause feelings of depression, or from the process of withdrawing from alcohol or other drugs.

Some research does examine the relationship between substance use and depression during pregnancy. Researchers estimate that six to 19 per cent of women use alcohol or illicit drugs at some time during pregnancy (Kelly et al., 2001). Substance use during pregnancy has been strongly associated with high EPDS scores (Pajulo et al., 2001a; Pajulo et al., 2001b). Additional research is required to understand perinatal mood disorders in women who use substances.

Women with PPD who use substances may be unlikely to seek treatment for fear of being judged by service providers or out of fear that child welfare authorities will apprehend the baby or older children. Women with current or past substance use problems may also have some particular issues when it comes to choice of treatment for PPD; those who endorse abstinence as their treatment goal may see antidepressants as another form of "substance use" to be avoided.

Paradoxically, pregnancy and the postpartum period may offer a window of opportunity for women who use substances to obtain treatment, as women who are depressed are more likely to seek treatment for substance use problems than are substance-dependent women without depression. Similarly, research shows that women's concerns about the dangers or effects of their substance use on their children spur them on to seek treatment (McMahon et al., 2002).

Substance use problems are significant health problems that may require attention by addiction specialists. However, all service providers have a role to play in detecting substance use.

STRATEGIES FOR WORKING WITH WOMEN WHO MAY BE USING SUBSTANCES

- Be aware of signs of problem substance use, which can be similar to symptoms of depression, such as:
  - agitation/irritability
  - mood swings
  - alienation and self-imposed social isolation
  - inability to keep up with responsibilities due to time spent seeking or obtaining substances (e.g., time spent away from home that the woman can't explain).

- Some health units/organizations may routinely screen for substance use. However, if this is not the case for your agency and you suspect someone has a substance use problem, you will need to follow up on this. Creating a non-judgmental context for asking questions about substance use is very important, as many mothers fear losing custody of their children if they indicate that they need help in this area (Poole & Isaac, 2001). There are a number of standardized screening tools for alcohol use, including the CAGE, the TWEAK and the Alcohol Use Disorder Identification Test (AUDIT) (Bradley et al., 1998). Also ask informally about use of alcohol or other substances, using questions such as the following:
  - Do you drink, smoke or use other substances to help you cope or relax?
  - [If yes] What substances are you using?
  - How often are you using [the substance]? Every day? Four or five times a week? Two or three times a week? Two to four times a month? [Ask for each substance used.]
  - Have you ever had a problem with drinking or drug use in the past?
  - How is your drinking/drug use affecting your ability to take care of yourself or the baby?

  Refer the woman for further assessment if she is using illicit recreational drugs or alcohol more than two or three times a week, and/or has had a problem in the past, and/or is reporting that her use is interfering with her ability to care for herself or her baby. Major urban centres have treatment programs specifically for women who are pregnant or parenting. (See Appendix D for a list of examples.) In other communities, you can refer women to their family doctor, another physician or mental health services. You may prefer not to leave the mother to make an appointment for herself (e.g., with her family doctor). And you should follow up with her to ensure that she has been able to access appropriate care.

- For more information about working with women who use substances, please refer to *The Hidden Majority: A Guidebook on Alcohol and Other Drug Issues for Counsellors Who Work with Women* (Addiction Research Foundation, 1996).

Women with Current and/or Past Experience of Abuse or Violence

Small studies of women seeking treatment for severe PPD have reported high rates of personal histories of childhood abuse (Buist & Janson, 2001). In one study of women surveyed upon admission to a mother-baby unit for PPD, 50 per cent of the sample reported childhood sexual abuse. Researchers have associated a history of physical or sexual abuse with particularly severe symptoms of depression and anxiety, as well as greater impairment of mother-infant attachment than that found in other women with PPD who have no history of sexual abuse.

Research suggests that approximately seven per cent of adult women and 22 per cent of adolescents experience physical abuse during pregnancy (Renker, 1999; Stewart & Cecutti, 1993). Researchers have associated prenatal physical abuse with both postpartum physical abuse and postpartum psychological distress (Stewart, 1994).

Physical, sexual and emotional abuse are serious clinical issues that are disturbingly common among women. A detailed discussion of the impact of violence on women's health is beyond the scope of this book; service providers may want to seek out other resources and training to help them address this important health issue.

STRATEGIES FOR WORKING WITH WOMEN WHO MAY HAVE EXPERIENCED VIOLENCE

- Inquire about current or past violence (as long as appropriate referral sources are available—see below). Normalize the process by indicating that you ask all clients these questions, and use a relaxed and straightforward tone of voice. Keep in mind that women may be reluctant to divulge their experiences of abuse: you may need to ask about abuse more than once over the duration of your clinical relationship. You can ask questions such as:
  - How is your relationship going?
  - Have you ever felt mistreated or harmed by someone you care about (such as a family member, partner or friend)?
- Keep in mind that symptoms or behaviours that appear to be dysfunctional could be coping strategies in the context of the overwhelming effects of interpersonal violence. Coping strategies that appear dysfunctional today might well have protected the woman from further harm in her past. An individual can form her sense of self in part around these coping mechanisms. Make every effort to understand the woman's emotional state in the context of her experiences.

- Be mindful that speaking about experiences of abuse or violence, particularly for the first time, can evoke feelings of extreme anxiety or distress, particularly for an individual who experienced threats of harm if she were to tell anyone about the abuse.
- Be sure to familiarize yourself with local referral options for women who are dealing with current or past abuse before asking screening questions. Many communities have 24-hour telephone help lines to offer support. (See Appendix D.) You may also want to prepare a list of local or regional mental health care providers/physicians who are experienced in counselling women who have experienced violence.
- For more information about working with women with histories of trauma, please refer to the CAMH publication *Bridging Responses* (Haskell, 2001).

PPD in Aboriginal Women

To the authors' knowledge, no research has specifically addressed the prevalence of, or risk factors for, PPD among Canadian Aboriginal women. The term *Aboriginal* refers to the indigenous people of Canada and their descendants, including First Nations, Inuit and Metis peoples. The Aboriginal community thus comprises many diverse groups, and each distinct Aboriginal community has unique values, issues and traditions with respect to health and healing (Reading, 2003).

Aboriginal people in Canada have worse overall health status than most other Canadians. A recent Health Canada report found that only 38 per cent of First Nations people in Ontario reported very good or excellent health, compared with 61 per cent of all Canadians. In terms of mental health, Health Canada reports that First Nations people lost three times as many years of life to suicide than did other Canadians (Grace, 2003). These health disparities are particularly true of Aboriginal women. Aboriginal women are more likely than women in the general Canadian population to die from cirrhosis or other alcohol-related complication, suicide or homicide (Mao et al., 1992). Variables linked to depression in non-Aboriginal women, including substance use and physical and sexual violence, occur more commonly in Aboriginal women than in the rest of the Canadian population (MacMillan et al., 2003).

Researchers largely attribute the poor health of Aboriginal people in Canada to poverty and the poor quality of life many of them face. Socio-economic hardship, violence and discrimination are likely to put Aboriginal women at risk for depression throughout their lives, including in the perinatal period.

Aboriginal women may also face significant isolation. Those living on reserves or in remote communities must sometimes leave their communities to give birth, perhaps for several weeks in the case of high-risk pregnancies, because the required medical facilities/services are not available in their own communities. Leaving the community often means that they will lack practical and emotional support. Kinship bonds may also have been disrupted when family members were forced to leave their communities to attend residential schools or to be adopted outside the Aboriginal community.

Access to culturally appropriate care, particularly for women who are not fluent in English (or French, depending upon the region), can be difficult. Aboriginal women may find it hard to access prenatal classes, parenting classes or postpartum follow-up resources, since those available may not be sensitive to Aboriginal culture and history. Similarly, service providers may find it difficult to educate family or community members about PPD if they do not speak English or French.

STRATEGIES FOR WORKING WITH ABORIGINAL WOMEN

- Very little is known about rates of PPD in Aboriginal women or effective strategies for assessing and treating this group. More research about and services for Aboriginal women with PPD are urgently needed. Take a holistic approach to treatment. Consult with the family and community elders, and refer Aboriginal women to appropriate social and/or other medical services as indicated. Take care to be knowledgeable about and respectful of Aboriginal traditions and beliefs.

PPD in Adolescent and Single Mothers

Research has identified high rates of PPD in both adolescent and unmarried mothers. Several studies have linked single status with symptoms of PPD (Lane et al., 1997; Pfost et al., 1990; Schaper et al., 1994; Hiscock & Wake, 2001). Studies examining the prevalence of postpartum major and minor depression in adolescent samples have reported rates as high as 26 per cent (Troutman & Cutrona, 1990).

Certain risk factors for PPD are likely to be more common in adolescent and single mothers than among other women of child-bearing age, in particular, lack of social support. Also, many adolescent and single mothers have unplanned and/or unwanted pregnancies. Social and economic factors, rather than maternal age alone, likely account for the increased risk for PPD and other adverse health outcomes in adolescent mothers (Logsdon, 2004).

STRATEGIES FOR WORKING WITH ADOLESCENT MOTHERS

- Find out what other workers or service providers are involved in her care, and get in touch with them if possible (observing client confidentiality) to ensure that you are not duplicating services or giving conflicting advice to the mother.
- Enlist the support of her family members and/or partner as much as is possible and appropriate.
- Treat each contact with an adolescent mother as though it could be your last. Because of the many barriers to care that adolescents face (e.g., lack of access to child care, transportation), they commonly miss appointments, so don't defer making important referrals or providing necessary advice and support.
- When making a referral to another service provider, consider attending the first appointment with the adolescent mother to facilitate her taking the referral.
- Where possible, refer to services (e.g., parenting education) that are directed toward adolescents and will address their unique needs.

STRATEGIES FOR WORKING WITH SINGLE MOTHERS

- Help the mother to think creatively about the people who can make up her support network. For example, is there a favourite aunt or family friend who might be willing to provide occasional help with baby care or housework?
- Provide information and encouragement to enable her to build up a support network of other mothers who may also be parenting with little support. This might include referral to community mothers' groups, family resource centres or Mother Goose programs. Many new mothers will neither be aware that these programs exist nor know how to access them.
- Cover the costs of transportation and child care whenever possible.
- Offer referrals to employment, education, housing and other social services as needed.

PPD in Lesbian and Bisexual Mothers

More and more women in same-sex relationships are now choosing to parent: a 1996 Canadian study found that 30 per cent of lesbians surveyed had or planned to have children (Moran, 1996). Although mothers parenting in same-sex versus opposite-sex relationships likely share many of the fundamental aspects of the transition to parenthood, lesbian and **bisexual** mothers may differ from heterosexual parents in many ways that could influence their risk for PPD.

Overall, studies report higher rates of past psychiatric disturbances among lesbian, gay and bisexual people than in heterosexual populations. Researchers have attributed these high rates to the stresses faced by lesbian, gay and bisexual people (and others who do not identify as heterosexual, including transgender and transsexual people) as a result of social discrimination (Meyer, 2003). However, history of depression is a strong risk factor for PPD, and lesbian and bisexual women as a group may be more likely than heterosexual women to have had depressive episodes.

Lesbian and bisexual mothers face other factors that could contribute to their risk for PPD; these factors might include lack of support from the family of origin (if the mother has not disclosed her sexual orientation to family, or if family are disapproving), social disapproval of lesbian parenthood, chronic stress associated with **homophobia** (fear of people who are, or are presumed to be, homosexual) and **heterosexism** (the assumption that everyone is, or should be, heterosexual) from family, strangers and those working in the health care system (Epstein, 2002).

Other variables, however, may protect lesbian and bisexual mothers from PPD. Unplanned pregnancies are rare among lesbians. In addition, many studies have demonstrated that same-sex couples are much more likely than their heterosexual counterparts to share child-care tasks equitably (Vanfraussen et al., 2003). Since lack of partner support is a risk factor for PPD, equal sharing of child-care labour may offer some protection from PPD.

STRATEGIES FOR WORKING WITH LESBIAN AND BISEXUAL MOTHERS

- Avoid making assumptions about the woman's sexual orientation. Using gender-neutral language when referring to a partner may help to create an atmosphere in which the mother feels comfortable disclosing her sexual orientation. For more information about using appropriate language when talking to women about sexual orientation, refer to the CAMH publication *Asking the Right Questions 2: Talking with clients about sexual orientation and gender identity in mental health, counselling and addiction settings (Barbara & Doctor, 2004)*.
- Check your own biases and assumptions about lesbianism. Socialization has led many of us to believe that lesbians are not or should not be mothers. Your internalized (and certainly explicit) homophobia or heterosexism will filter through and affect the kind of care provided, even in subtle ways.
- Find out who is in the woman's support network: some women may be estranged from families of origin but have a supportive community of friends.
- Support from other lesbian and bisexual parents can help. In small communities where this may not be available, women may be able to access e-mail or Internet support (e.g., familypride.uwo.ca/; www.fsatoronto.com/programs/fsaprograms/davekelley/lgbtparenting.html).

Depression in Adoptive Mothers

Little research has examined the emotional experiences of women in the post-adoption period; however, studies have found evidence that some adoptive women do experience depression during the first months as a parent.

Historical literature on PPD includes a few case reports of women who experienced episodes of depression shortly after adoption (Melges, 1968; Victoroff, 1952). Another study compared the lifetime prevalence of psychiatric illness among women who had adopted children to women who had both adopted and biological children. Women in the group with both adoptive and biological children were twice as likely to report having an episode of depression within 12 months of birth or adoption (Dean et al., 1995). However, in the group of women who had children only through adoption, eight per cent reported experiencing an episode of depression within 12 months of the adoption.

In one study, 19 adoptive mothers completed the EPDS, and thought back to how they were feeling in the early post-adoption period. Although this research design has some flaws (in particular, uncertainty about how accurately women can recall how they were feeling up to five years ago), interestingly, 32 per cent of mothers had scores greater than or equal to 12 on the EPDS (Gair, 1999). Most of these women attributed their distress to severe sleep disruption and/or colicky babies, and many of them used the words "postnatal depression" to describe their experiences.

Service providers and mothers themselves may assume that adoption is not associated with depression, since only women who are clearly looking forward to becoming mothers undertake adoption. However, as a result of their great desire to have children, these women may have a particularly idealized expectation of motherhood, and so may be vulnerable to depression when things are not as they had expected, or when the child has special needs. (This same situation may also apply to women who undergo fertility procedures to achieve pregnancy.)

Adoptive mothers may face some unique issues. For example, some may be coming to terms with their own infertility or the lack of ancestral ties with their children. The adoption process itself can be intrusive and stressful. Other women may worry that their children will face difficulties as a result of disruptions in parental attachment or lack of breastfeeding (reviewed in Gair, 1999). On the other hand, adoptive mothers tend to be somewhat older than biological mothers, and therefore perhaps more adept at coping with life stress; they tend to be financially secure; and they are often in a stable relationship—factors that some have suggested could help protect adoptive mothers (Levy-Shiff et al., 1990).

STRATEGIES FOR WORKING WITH ADOPTIVE MOTHERS

- Be aware that mothers who adopt also face significant physical and emotional stress, particularly after adopting an infant. If possible, connect them with supports that can address the primary causes of their distress (e.g., involving the partner or other support people to enable the mother to get some uninterrupted sleep; referral to a counsellor or **psychologist** if she is dealing with issues related to infertility).
- Educate mothers and their families about the myths of motherhood (Chapter 9). Women who adopt, in particular, may feel they cannot or should not have any negative emotions related to their babies.
- Help women to connect with other mothers who have adopted if they desire to do so. (See Appendix D.)

Women with Chronic Mental Illness or Other Disabilities

Health professionals need to differentiate between women with PPD and women with chronic mental illnesses, such as severe depression and schizophrenia. For some women with PPD, the postpartum episode is their first experience with depression. As described in Chapter 5, when treated promptly and appropriately, most women with PPD will make a full recovery. In contrast, for women with chronic mental illness such as schizophrenia or bipolar disorder, the disease recurs throughout their lives, and in many cases, is severe. It generally has a significant impact on a woman's ability to function at work, socially and as a parent. (See Gopfert et al., 2004 for more information on parents with mental health disorders.)

Women with severe mental illness appear to be as likely as other women to have children but, in many cases, do not retain full custody of their children (Nicholson et al., 1998). Research on mothers with severe mental illness has highlighted the emotional and economic or practical support available to them in early parenthood as key issues that determine how successfully they will be able to parent (Mowbray et al., 1995). However, fear of custody loss can prevent women from asking for the support they need (Nicholson et al., 1998).

In focus groups with women with severe mental illness, mothers and their caregivers identified four themes that predominated in their parenting experiences (Nicholson et al., 1998):

- *Stigma associated with their illness.* Many people assume that women with mental illness are not capable of caring for a child, and as a result, these mothers feel that they constantly need to prove themselves (in contrast to mothers without disabilities, whom everyone presumes to be good parents until proven otherwise).

- *A tendency to evaluate themselves against unrealistic expectations.* Mothers may assume that even "normal" bad behaviour in their children somehow results from their illness. Either the mothers themselves or those around them may take any feelings of stress or dissatisfaction with motherhood as a signal that they are not good parents.
- *Difficulty balancing their children's best interest against their own.* For mothers with mental illness, their own **self-care** may directly conflict with the needs of their children; for example, a mother may need to take a medication that slows her ability to respond to her children, or she may need to schedule numerous medical appointments during hours when she feels she should be available to her children.
- *Concern about ability to maintain contact with and custody of their children.* Women may find this particularly difficult through periods of hospitalization, or as a result of voluntary temporary care, involuntary removal by child protection services, or divorce.

Researchers and clinicians have noted that, like the general population of women, women with mental illness vary in parenting skill, and many mothers with mental illness parent very capably.

Women with other forms of disability, including sensory, physical or learning disabilities, face many of the same issues as mothers with chronic mental illnesses. In particular, they must deal with other people assuming that they are unfit parents, with a lack of appropriate support and with difficulties balancing their own needs with those of their children (Kelley et al., 1997; Llewellyn & McConnell, 2002). Research suggests that although parents with disabilities may have significant barriers to overcome, many develop substitute skills that enable them to cope effectively with their children's needs (Sheerin, 1998). Service providers can be instrumental in helping women with disabilities to develop helpful parenting skills and coping techniques.

STRATEGIES FOR WORKING WITH MOTHERS WITH CHRONIC MENTAL ILLNESS OR OTHER DISABILITIES

- Remember that many women with chronic mental illness and other disabilities will care for their children effectively, even when the illness or disability is severe.
- Reassure mothers about the normal range of child behaviour and parenting stress. This may help to alleviate guilt arising from the belief that their disability has "caused" all of their child's problems or that their feelings of being overwhelmed mean that they are inadequate parents.
- Work with each mother individually to determine her parenting skills and needs. Like women without disabilities, parenting skills and needs will vary from person to person.
- Once you have carefully assessed a mother's needs, you can help to connect her with the specific services or resources she needs (e.g., parenting education, practical or financial support).
- Ensure care co-ordination, so that the mother does not feel overwhelmed by multi-agency involvement and so services are not duplicated.

Summary

Some examples of populations that may have unique mental health needs during the perinatal period include:
- women of diverse ethnocultural origins, and particularly immigrant and refugee women
- women from rural or remote communities
- women who use alcohol and other substances
- women who have experienced physical or sexual abuse
- Aboriginal women
- adolescent and single mothers
- lesbian mothers
- adoptive mothers
- women with chronic mental illnesses or other disabilities.

Service providers working with diverse populations should:
- Be prepared to provide referral to language, employment, housing and other social services as required.
- Educate yourself as much as possible about the particular needs and issues of the women who use your services.
- Do not rely exclusively on English-language, or even translated, screening tools, but ask some general questions such as the following: "How have you been feeling?" "How have you been sleeping?" "How has your appetite been?" "Is there anything you have been worrying about?"
- Avoid making false assumptions. Each woman brings a unique set of beliefs and experiences to her childbirth experience, regardless of her ethnocultural background, marital status or sexual orientation. Ask women what issues are important to them, rather than assuming that you know.
- If a woman needs intervention, seek out specialized services (developed to meet the unique needs of a specific population) if available and if she is interested in them. Women may benefit in particular from group treatment or support when their fellow group members share similar experiences and beliefs.

9
Self-Care Strategies for Postpartum Women

Can self-care play a role in postpartum depression?

What self-care strategies can service providers recommend to postpartum women?

This chapter provides some simple **self-care** strategies that mothers may find helpful during the postpartum period. However, the strategies suggested here will not in any way suffice as treatment for depression, nor enable a woman with **postpartum depression (PPD)** to recover. Rather, the suggestions provided should serve as adjuncts to appropriate medical and/or psychological treatment for PPD. In conjunction with this treatment, self-care strategies may help a woman with PPD to regain a sense of control over her situation and empower her to take the necessary steps toward recovery.

A mother with depression may not, at first, feel well enough to do many of the self-care activities listed here. After treatment begins to take effect, however, she will have more and more energy, and will gradually be able to initiate self-care. Service providers should encourage women to use whichever strategies they think might help most.

Developing Realistic Expectations about Motherhood

As mentioned in Chapter 3, our society has idealized images about what motherhood is like. In particular, parenting magazines, books and other media suggest that any feelings of sadness, anxiety or anger are abnormal for a mother of a new baby. In reality, no mother of an infant will be as happy, as organized or as relaxed as the woman on the cover of the parenting magazine appears to be.

Many mothers will compare themselves to female relatives or friends who seem to have managed motherhood perfectly, and inevitably feel that there is something wrong with them if they can't manage as easily. These comparisons, too, help to reinforce the myths about motherhood.

Common myths about motherhood

- Giving birth is an "exclusively" positive and happy event in a woman's life.
- Mothers should be "superwomen": perfect mothers, perfect wives, perfect homemakers and accomplished career women all at the same time.
- Being a mother is a totally fulfilling experience for all women.
- Mothers have intuitive, natural, built-in maternal instincts and know immediately how to care for babies.
- Mothers enjoy all of the work associated with caring for a baby.
- Mothers feel loving toward their infants at all times, no matter what.
- Mothers are tireless, selfless and unconditionally giving of themselves.
- Mothers never get angry or irritable, and have unending patience.
- Mothers shouldn't need help caring for their babies.

Health care workers can help women identify and challenge misleading myths about motherhood so that they can build self-esteem and confidence in their capacity to parent. In reality, being a mother is hard work. As with any job involving high demand but little control over one's schedule, it is easy to feel burned out at times.

Getting As Much Sleep and Rest As Possible

Depending on how long labour and delivery take, most mothers go through a few days during and immediately following the baby's birth when they get little or no sleep. Even after the first few days, women caring for a new baby are likely to have their nighttime sleep interrupted by frequent awakenings to feed their baby. Considering all the sleep disruptions, most mothers not surprisingly feel perpetually tired or exhausted during the first weeks after giving birth.

Some researchers believe that sleep deprivation can trigger symptoms of anxiety, depression or even **psychosis** in women who have a number of the risk factors described in Chapter 2 (Sharma & Mazmanian, 2003). At the Women's Health Concerns Clinic at St. Joseph's Healthcare, Hamilton, Ontario, staff members focus much attention on attempting to reduce sleep deprivation in women who are at risk of developing PPD. Staff at the Women's Health Concerns Clinic recommend, as part of that care, many of the strategies included in this section.

STRATEGIES FOR CATCHING UP ON SLEEP

Getting sleep during a postpartum hospital stay

Many mothers feel as though they are unable to rest during their hospital stay, due to disruptions associated with care from hospital staff, other patients in the same room and visitors. To minimize disruptions, mothers can tell caregivers when they are trying to rest and ask not to be disturbed for a while.

Tips for mothers:
- You can help keep things quiet in your hospital room by putting meal trays outside the door when you've finished eating, and by letting caregivers know when you are resting and do not wish to be disturbed.
- Attach a "do not disturb" sign to the door of your room when you are trying to rest, so that visitors and caregivers will know you are sleeping.

Limiting visitors

Family and friends will naturally be curious and excited to meet the new baby, and the mother may be delighted to introduce her baby to the important people in her life. However, a constant flow of visitors can add to the stress and exhaustion of the early postpartum period. Family—particularly partners—can support mothers by discouraging visitors from coming at inconvenient times. They can also encourage mothers to consider their own need for rest and quiet.

If women feel uncomfortable about telling people when they should or should not visit, they can ask their support people (partner, parents, relatives) to help in arranging visits at a convenient time. New mothers can also ask visitors to be flexible and allow them to cancel at the last minute if they are feeling tired and not up to seeing anyone.

> **Tips for mothers:**
> - You may want to plan an "open house" when everyone can come meet the baby at once. Before giving birth, give your family and friends an idea when you would like them to visit. You might suggest intervals for visits that you find are convenient for you and the baby, for example, from 2:00 p.m. to 3:00 p.m. Encourage people to come after the first week postpartum.
> - If you find that people do not always respect your wishes about when you would like them to visit, your partner and/or family members can let visitors know that you are resting and ask them to come at another time.
> - Try putting a "do not disturb" sign beside the doorbell and unplug the telephone when you want to take a nap.

Eating Well

Mothers who are home alone with a new baby during the day may find it difficult, if not impossible, to make time to prepare (or even to eat) meals. Yet a new mother can take some steps to provide nourishing food for herself. Being thoughtful about nutrition is a positive form of self-care.

First, she can ask others to help with food preparation, if they are willing. Visitors could come at mealtime and bring along enough food for everyone. The new mother could invite relatives and friends to give a one-dish meal that is ready to freeze as a welcome gift. Suggestions for this type of gift include a casserole, a hearty soup, a stew or a curry. Alternatively, healthy frozen entrees are available at supermarkets, and the new mother could buy these to have on hand when cooking seems like too much of a chore.

Mothers can take a few minutes during the baby's morning nap or when the baby goes down at night to prepare small meals or snacks for themselves for the coming day. Mothers can eat nutritious, high-energy snack foods while feeding the baby.

Mothers, especially those who are breastfeeding, should stay well hydrated. Dehydration can exacerbate feelings of low energy. Mothers should drink before they are thirsty, as thirst is an early sign of dehydration. A mother is drinking enough when her urine is pale yellow.

Tips for mothers:

Finger foods that mothers can snack on while feeding the baby:

• cut-up fresh fruit	• dried fruit	• hard-boiled eggs
• trail mix*	• muffins	• cornbread
• chapati	• dhal or naan breads	• Chinese buns
• pita bread with hummus	• crackers with cheese	• toast and peanut butter**

Examples of foods to keep ready-to-eat in the refrigerator:

• yogourt	• leftover rice and peas	• roti
• soup or stew	• curry	• pasta salad

Keep bottles of water, milk or pure fruit juice handy. Limit coffee with caffeine to no more than two mugs (250 mL/8 oz.) per day. Many women find tea a comforting drink and it is lower in caffeine than coffee. Herbal teas are caffeine-free. If you use alcohol, you should limit it to an occasional drink, especially if you are breastfeeding.

* Breastfeeding mothers who have a family history of allergies should avoid peanuts and discuss with their doctor whether they should avoid other foods.

Getting Exercise

Moderate exercise in the postpartum period can improve overall energy levels, relieve stress and muscle tension, improve muscle strength needed to carry and feed the baby, and help a woman's body recover more quickly from pregnancy and childbirth.

Tips for mothers:

• The process of returning to or beginning physical activity after giving birth varies from individual to individual. If you had a healthy, uncomplicated pregnancy and delivery, and feel comfortable, you can begin a mild exercise program immediately. Light intensity activities may include stretching, walking and pelvic floor exercises. If you had a Caesarean birth or complications during your pregnancy or delivery, consult your doctor or other health care provider before resuming physical activity.

• Be on the lookout for fitness or yoga classes in your community. Specific postpartum classes will usually welcome your baby—the baby can either participate with you (babies make great free weights), or child care may be available. These classes also provide a great opportunity to meet other mothers of young babies in your area.

> **Tips for mothers: (continued)**
> - Brisk walks with the baby in a stroller are great exercise, since the stroller provides some extra resistance. In the winter or bad weather, consider taking the baby for a walk around your nearest shopping mall; or, if you live in a community without an appropriate place for indoor walking, dress yourself and the baby up warmly and go for shorter periods of time, or try another form of exercise (e.g., exercise videos).
> - Keep safe when being active. If physical activity causes any pain or you experience heavy bleeding, stop the activity and talk to your doctor or other health care provider. Remember to drink enough when being active.
> - If you are breastfeeding, you may find that wearing two bras helps to stabilize your breasts.

Developing and Taking Advantage of a Support Network

Given the many demands of a newborn, many mothers spend most of the day at home alone with their children, often having little or no contact with other adults. Consequently, mothers commonly feel trapped and lonely.

Mothers alone with a new baby may feel isolated, especially during bad weather, when it might not seem worth the effort of bundling up to face the cold or heat. Social isolation can negatively affect the mother's mood and may exacerbate depression, particularly if she is accustomed to socializing regularly with other adults (e.g., at work, at the gym, for leisure activities).

TALKING TO OTHER MOTHERS OF NEW BABIES

One of the best ways for women to deconstruct the myths about motherhood (see page 108) is to talk to other mothers about their experiences. Mothers who are lucky enough to have family and friends with young children may have the opportunity to do this through informal social networks. For mothers who don't have an existing support network of new parents, joining a group that puts mothers in touch with each other may help them to feel less alone, and to recognize that many other mothers face similar challenges and struggles.

However, women who are depressed may find a neighbourhood mothers' group intimidating or upsetting: women with depression may feel that the other members of the group seem to be coping better than they are, exacerbating their sense of guilt and inadequacy. In this case, women may find PPD-specific groups a better choice. Although these groups are harder to find, they do exist in many areas. (See Directories of PPD Support Groups in the list of Resources at the end of this guide, page 158.)

Tips for mothers:

- Join a group for mothers of new babies. Many public health units and community groups or agencies organize weekly groups for mothers. (See Appendix D, page 156.) You can also try organizing your own informal mothers' group by arranging to meet with family and friends who have young children.
- Ask your support people to help you get some time outside the house or apartment without the baby. For example, meet a friend for lunch or to go shopping while someone else watches the baby.
- If getting out of the house or apartment just seems too overwhelming, try starting out by using the telephone or e-mail to re-establish social contacts.

INVOLVING THE PARTNER AS MUCH AS POSSIBLE

For women with supportive partners, the partner will probably be as keen as the mother is to learn how to be a good parent. A mother can take advantage of the partner's willingness to help with all and any tasks, such as diaper changes, settling or calming the baby, feeds and post-feed burping, and household chores.

Alone, or "quality," time for the partner and newborn can help the two of them bond, and gives the mother a much-needed chance to rest and have time for herself.

Tips for mothers:

- You may think you know best how to handle, feed and otherwise care for your new baby. When you see your partner doing things differently, you might be tempted to try and take over or suggest a better way to do things. Resist this temptation; your baby needs to learn how it feels to be handled by different people. Otherwise, down the road, your child may only settle with you, which only makes it harder for others to help out when needed.
- If you find yourself feeling anxious or hovering over your partner when he or she is caring for the baby, you will probably both feel better if you leave the room or home.

ASKING OTHER SUPPORT PEOPLE FOR HELP

Mothers often feel guilty or embarrassed about asking for help because they may feel they shouldn't need it. Looking after a new baby is hard work, and mothers can use all possible assistance. Mothers may want to make a list of names and telephone numbers to have for situations when they might require or want some help.

Tips for mothers:

- When friends or family members offer to help, take advantage of the offer. Tell them exactly what they can do to help (e.g., bring over dinner, do a load of laundry, watch the baby while you have a nap or take a bath) and when you would like them to do these things.
- If someone is available to look after the baby, take advantage of the time to rest, and resist the temptation to do housework. (The mess will still be there when you get up from your nap, but you may not have another chance to catch up on the missed sleep.)
- When a support person is available to take care of the baby, take advantage of the opportunity to get out on your own for some quiet time to rejuvenate, to enjoy the company of other adults or to do whatever else you feel like at the time.

Heeding the Warning Signs of Stress and Responding Appropriately

An important aspect of self-care is becoming familiar with your limits and warning signs: signals that suggest you are feeling overwhelmed, stressed and need a break. Service providers should encourage mothers to watch for their own triggers (i.e., people or activities that tend to make them feel stressed or unhappy), as well as warning signs that they may become anxious or down if they continue what they are doing.

LISTENING TO SIGNALS

Service providers should urge a woman to listen to her own signals, which may include:

- the shakes, jitteriness
- back pain
- door slamming
- raised voice, sarcasm
- rejections or obstinate refusals of help
- clenched jaw, palpitations
- holding the breath
- noises sounding louder than usual
- distressing thoughts (e.g., "I can't stand this," or "I'm not coping" or "I need help.")
- muddled or confused mindset
- irritability or numbness
- decreased confidence in one's abilities (e.g., as a mother)
- indecisiveness, unable to make decisions.

CALMING ACTIVITIES

Service providers should urge new mothers to experiment with activities that may be calming when triggers or warning signs indicate that they are starting to feel overwhelmed.

> **Tips for mothers:**
> - Take a shower or bath.
> - Do deep breathing—focus attention on breathing, rather than on negative thoughts.
> - Telephone a friend or caregiver.
> - Tell yourself: "It will be all right. I am doing the best I can at the moment."
> - Try positive self-statements: "I can do this" or "You can get through this."
> - Relax tense muscles.
> - Remind yourself that you are not alone; others are in the same situation.

If a mother continues to feel overwhelmed or anxious when using these simple strategies, or if the feelings persist, the woman may require medical and/or psychological treatment. (Please refer to Chapter 6.)

Summary

Self-care is not a substitute for appropriate medical or psychological treatment. However, self-care strategies should be considered as part of a comprehensive treatment plan. These strategies may empower a woman to take some of the necessary steps toward her recovery.

Useful self-care strategies for all postpartum women include:
- recognizing unrealistic expectations about what motherhood might be like
- getting as much rest as possible: limiting visitors, letting others know when she is resting
- asking support people for help preparing food, caring for the baby, doing housework
- accepting help that support people, including the partner, may offer
- eating well: preparing one-dish meals, encouraging visitors to bring food, stocking up on healthy, high-energy snacks
- getting moderate exercise: taking it slow, going for walks with the baby, postpartum fitness classes
- building a strong support network: getting out of the house as much as possible, making an effort to meet other mothers with new babies, keeping in touch with family and friends

10

Case Studies

This section provides some sample cases of women presenting for postpartum care who are reporting symptoms that could indicate **postpartum depression (PPD)**. Based on the information provided, consider the following questions: Are the new mother's problems attributable to PPD, or another more or less serious condition? What additional information would you like to have before deciding how to proceed? And what, if anything, would you do to help address the new mother's concerns? The authors provide suggestions following each case.

Case #1: Lucy

Lucy is a 29-year-old married woman who has lived in Toronto for the past 10 years. She is visiting your community drop-in program for the first time since having her first child, a healthy baby boy, one week ago.

Lucy's husband has returned to work after taking a couple of days off after the birth. He works at a factory, with 12-hour shifts, including some night shifts. Most of Lucy's family live in Toronto and have been dropping by to visit periodically since the baby was born.

When asked, Lucy reports that in the past few days, she has been feeling very emotional and cries easily. She has slept little as a result of caring for the baby through the night, and has difficulty concentrating and making simple decisions. She also reports feeling very worried about her son's health, and is concerned that she is not caring for him as well as she should. She is tearful during the interview but her mood appears to lift somewhat when her son requires her attention.

QUESTIONS TO ASK

- How long has Lucy been feeling this way? (Need to determine if symptoms began postpartum and could be the "blues," or whether she may have been depressed during the pregnancy.)
- Has Lucy ever felt this way in the past?

Lucy reports that she felt well throughout her pregnancy and that these symptoms seemed to begin within a few days of giving birth. She does not recall ever feeling this sad or tearful before.

STRATEGIES AND RECOMMENDATIONS

- Since Lucy just gave birth one week ago, she is more likely experiencing the "baby blues" than PPD. Reassure Lucy that these feelings are not uncommon, and that they are not signs that she is somehow abnormal or a bad mother.
- Encourage her to use any available supports, including her family, to help her get consecutive hours of sleep, which will likely ease some of her symptoms. Is there someone she can ask to watch the baby for her for a couple of hours in the afternoon? What about someone to help with the baby at night? If it is financially possible, perhaps her husband could take a few additional days off work.
- Request that she return in one to two weeks for follow-up, to ensure that the blues are not masking PPD or do not develop into PPD. If the symptoms worsen before her follow-up appointment, encourage her to seek medical advice or call her local public health department.

Case #2: Leila

Leila is a 32-year-old married woman who immigrated to Vancouver from Central America with her husband one year ago. Her first language is Spanish and she has difficulty communicating in English. She visits your Early Years Centre with her six-month-old son, her only child.

Leila has none of her own family in Canada, but her husband's parents and brother are in Vancouver. For financial reasons, none of her family members have been able to visit her since the baby was born. Her husband works long hours in construction, but Leila describes him as being very supportive and a good father. She has met a few acquaintances through her husband's co-workers, but reports that she has no close friends in Canada.

When asked, Leila reports feeling "not like herself." When you probe further, she reveals that she sleeps very little even now that her son is sleeping through the night, has spells of crying and feels constantly worried about even minor things.

When you inquire about her support network, Leila says she feels very lonely and is disappointed that she has no one to visit her and her new baby. In the interview, she appears restless and easily distracted.

QUESTIONS TO ASK

- Has Leila ever felt this way in the past?
- Does she have anyone who is helping her with the baby while she is at home during the day?

When asked, Leila reports that she had symptoms similar to these when her father died about 10 years ago. She explains that she does not have help with the baby, because she doesn't know many people in Canada.

You decide to administer a Spanish translation of the **Edinburgh Postnatal Depression Scale (EPDS)**, and find that Leila has a total score of 14, with a score of zero on item 10 of the EPDS—meaning that she does not endorse thoughts of harming herself.

STRATEGIES AND RECOMMENDATIONS

- Leila's total EPDS score is in the range of probable depression, although you should interpret these results cautiously since the validity of the Spanish translation is not well established. Explain to Leila that she may have PPD and educate her about the condition. Provide as much material in Spanish as possible.
- Consider Leila's risk for PPD: she reports some risk factors for PPD, including lack of social support and a previous episode of depression.
- If she has experienced symptoms for two weeks or more, refer Leila to her family doctor or mental health professional to confirm a diagnosis of PPD and begin treatment. (See Figure 6–1 on page 63.) Leila will need to be monitored in case her symptoms worsen or she develops suicidal thoughts. Recommend that she return to the clinic in one to two weeks.
- Leila's symptoms may also respond to psychosocial interventions, such as encouraging her husband to take some time away from work to help her or encouraging her to attend mother-baby groups. (You can help by checking with Spanish community organizations for mother-baby groups conducted in Spanish.)

Case #3: Maryann

An obstetrician has referred Maryann, age 32, for a public health home visit. According to the doctor's referral note, Maryann has felt exhausted and unwell since her difficult delivery eight weeks ago. At her six-week postpartum checkup with the obstetrician, she described headaches, fatigue, stomach pains and low mood. She was also worried about her baby's health, as she thought he looked sick, although the doctor assured her the baby was fine.

The obstetrician's examination revealed no physical health problems. Instead of feeling relieved, Maryann burst into tears and asked, "Then how come I feel so rotten?" He reassured her that many new mothers have trouble adjusting and that when the baby began to sleep through the night she would likely feel better. He also suggested that she might be feeling stressed as a result of her recent move to Ottawa from Alberta.

QUESTIONS TO ASK

• Has Maryann ever felt this way before?
• Who does she have to support her in Ottawa?

Maryann reports two previous episodes of depression unrelated to pregnancy, at ages 18 and 26. She reports that she misses support from her friends and family in Alberta, and has made very few social connections since she has been in Ottawa. You note that Maryann has several risk factors for PPD, including previous depression, recent stress (move to Ottawa), poor social support and a difficult delivery.

After talking with her, you decide to administer the EPDS. Her score is 16, with a score of two on item 10 (thoughts of harming oneself). Recognizing that this EPDS score indicates probable depression, and in particular Maryann's risk for suicide, you contact her family doctor, who makes an urgent referral to a **psychiatrist**. In the meantime, you ensure that Maryann is not left by herself or alone with the baby.

You follow up with Maryann the next day, and she tells you that the psychiatrist determined that she has PPD. The psychiatrist reminded her that antidepressants had worked well for her previous depressions, prescribed them for her and arranged for weekly follow-up visits. You encourage Maryann to continue to take her medication and see the psychiatrist regularly, and also suggest that she attend a PPD support group in your area.

STRATEGIES AND RECOMMENDATIONS

- EPDS can be useful as a preliminary assessment of risk for suicide (score of greater than zero on item 10 requires further assessment). See pages 64 to 65 for more information about assessing suicidal risk. In Maryann's case, urgent referral for assessment was necessary.
- Suicidality is often a marker for severe depression that will require medical treatment. Knowing that Maryann has responded well to antidepressants in the past also helps determine specific treatment.
- Maryann has a limited social support network. Encourage her to develop a network of support in her new community. Refer her to a PPD peer support group that she can attend in conjunction with medical treatment. If support groups are not available in your community, consider telephone or Internet-based support.
- Follow up after a referral to a **family physician** or psychiatrist to ensure that Maryann was able to keep her appointment and that an appropriate health professional has initiated a treatment plan.

Case #4: Susan

Since Susan gave birth to a baby boy five days ago, her family has become increasingly concerned about her behaviour. Her partner has telephoned your local public health unit to discuss his concerns.

Susan appeared ecstatic after the birth, but now goes within a matter of hours from being happy to crying uncontrollably. She is becoming increasingly irritable, and argues with her mother and husband, which is completely out of character for her. She is rude to people and shows no concern if she hurts their feelings.

Susan has not slept much since the birth, claiming she doesn't need to, and that she has never felt more energized. She does housework in the middle of the night and rushes from one thing to another, never finishing a job before starting on something new. Her family cannot hold a conversation with her, as she jumps from topic to topic, and some of what she says does not make sense.

QUESTION TO ASK

- Has her family noticed Susan behaving unusually, or has she expressed bizarre beliefs?

Susan's partner notes that Susan has begun placing the baby's toys around his crib in a particular way, so that all the toys are facing toward him; she says that this will protect them all from harm. She lashes out at anyone who tries to move the toys, and no one can persuade her that this is unreasonable behaviour. She believes that people may hurt the baby because they know he is special. She intends to write a book about how to raise children, which she knows will be an international best-seller.

STRATEGIES AND RECOMMENDATIONS

- Susan is exhibiting important warning signs of **psychosis**: strange behaviour that is out of character for her, mood swings, and beliefs that others do not share and that no one can dissuade her from.
- Susan requires emergency referral to a psychiatrist for assessment of possible postpartum psychosis. She should not be left by herself or alone with the baby until this assessment occurs. You may want to find a family member or friend of Susan's who can look after the baby. If, in the rare case that you still have concerns about the baby's safety, you should contact the local child protection service.
- Susan may need to be admitted to a psychiatric hospital, and will likely start drug treatment (e.g., mood stabilizers or antipsychotics). Service providers should follow up to ensure that Susan is receiving appropriate care, and should keep Susan's family informed of the nature of her illness and the proposed treatment.

Case #5: Ghaada

Ghaada is a 22-year-old first-time mother who recently moved to Canada with her husband, Jameel, from South Asia. Three weeks ago, she gave birth to a healthy baby girl. Ghaada's extended family lives in her homeland. Her husband tries to provide assistance, but she primarily takes care of the baby herself. Frequently, Ghaada is overwhelmed and has little time to eat or sleep. She also finds herself crying, as she doubts her ability to be a good mother. She did not realize that motherhood would be such a struggle, and expected it to be a joyful time in her life. She does not let her husband know that she is experiencing difficulties, and tries to maintain the home in the same condition as she did before the baby was born.

QUESTION TO ASK

• If you were in your home country, how would your experience of having a new baby be different?

Ghaada explains that a traditional postpartum practice in her culture is for the mother of the woman who has given birth, as well as other female relatives, to give additional support for the first 40 days postpartum. She notes that she misses her mother and other relatives who would have taken part in this custom, and she feels that there is no one in Canada who can fill their role for her.

You explain to Ghaada that she might be experiencing PPD. She is surprised, and says that no one in her family has ever experienced PPD before. She suggests that what she is experiencing is a normal part of motherhood, and she would not be having these difficulties if her mother were staying with her. She also says that she has just seen her baby's pediatrician and he didn't indicate that he thought she was experiencing PPD. She is concerned about what her husband and family would think of this diagnosis.

STRATEGIES AND RECOMMENDATIONS

• Ghaada is concerned about **stigmatization**, especially from her family members. You may be able to help by giving Ghaada and her family members information about PPD, in their first language if possible. Explain that PPD is a medical condition like any other, and may require treatment.

• If Ghaada's symptoms persist for two weeks or more, a physician should assess her to determine whether or not she requires treatment for PPD. In any case, you should follow up to ensure that she receives appropriate care and that her symptoms do not worsen.

• Ghaada may be experiencing acculturative stress related to adapting to a new culture during a time that carries special meaning in her home culture. Encourage her to take up opportunities to meet other new mothers from the same cultural group (e.g., peer support groups).

Case #6: Linda

Linda is a 35-year-old mother who recently gave birth to her third child, a boy. Her other children are aged six and three. Linda lives with her husband, Scott, and her children on a farm in southwestern Ontario. Linda's family live in Western Canada and she sees them very infrequently, although she has regular telephone contact with her sister. Scott's family lives close by. However, Linda has had ongoing difficulties in her relationship with her in-laws since she and Scott married eight years ago.

Over the last two weeks, Linda has been feeling very low, and has been frequently crying for no reason that she can identify. She has been finding it difficult to cope with the needs of her children, and loses her temper easily. Linda is concerned about these feelings, since she did not experience anything like this following the birth of her other two children. Scott and his family have noticed the changes in Linda's mood and energy level, and have criticized her inability to keep up with the housework, child care and cooking responsibilities.

During your routine public health visit to Linda's home, you notice that she appears somewhat dishevelled and exhausted. Although she answers your questions, she responds with a simple yes or no, and seems unwilling to elaborate on how she has been feeling. You recognize that Linda may be having some problems and decide to probe further.

QUESTIONS TO ASK

- Noticing Linda's exhausted appearance, you comment that she looks tired and ask how she has been sleeping. (Discussing physical symptoms can sometimes lead to disclosure of psychological symptoms of depression.)
- You inquire about Linda's support network: Is there anyone who is helping her with the children? Who does she have to talk to?

Linda reveals that, for the last several weeks, she has been unable to sleep. She finds herself tossing and turning, even when all the children are sleeping. When asked if she has noticed any other changes, she mentions that she has been feeling short-tempered and overwhelmed by the children.

When asked about her support network, Linda reveals that she has had no help with the children. She has tried to talk to Scott about how she is feeling, but he has dismissed her concerns and is unwilling to take on any of the child-care responsibilities. Since Scott's family has always criticized her as a mother, Linda says that she would never consider asking them for help. Although Linda has a good relationship with her sister, she has found lately that she does not have the time or energy to keep in contact with her sister by telephone as she has done in the past.

FOLLOW-UP QUESTIONS

- Considering Scott's lack of support, you ask Linda whether or not she has had any difficulties in her marriage in the past. In particular, you ask whether or not Scott had been willing to help with child care for the other children.

With prompting and reassurance about confidentiality, Linda reveals that she and Scott have had problems in their relationship beginning well before the birth of this baby. She describes increasing problems communicating with each other, stating that Scott often spends long hours away from home, and seldom spends time with her or the children. She attributes these difficulties in part to her poor relationship with his family.

When probed, Linda reveals that she started having mood problems about six months ago, after a serious argument with Scott that resulted in him leaving home for a few days. She implies that her most recent pregnancy was unplanned, and that this unplanned pregnancy may have escalated their previous difficulties.

STRATEGIES AND RECOMMENDATIONS

- Although Linda's difficulties are happening in a postpartum context, your discussion reveals that they are most likely due to the relationship difficulties. Her lack of practical and emotional support is likely contributing to her sense of isolation, since she has no one with whom she feels she can discuss these difficulties. The relationship problems and lack of support would be appropriate targets for intervention.
- Counselling (individual or preferably couple) may help begin to address some of the problems in Linda's relationship with Scott. Depending on Linda's ability to pay for services, consider making a referral to counselling services in a nearby community.
- To address Linda's lack of support:
  - Suggest that she reconnect with her sister, who has provided a good source of emotional support in the past. Perhaps structured contact (e.g., weekly calls at a previously arranged time) would help build Linda's confidence in making use of this resource. If possible, encourage Linda to visit her sister, or have her sister visit her, as this might help lift her mood.
  - Suggest that she connect with any existing resources for mothers in her community (e.g., drop-in or library programs) to expand her support network. If she is unable to access programs for new mothers, perhaps she can make use of any telephone or Internet support that is available in surrounding communities.
  - Encourage Linda to identify people in her surrounding community who have offered support in the past or who might be willing to offer support. Remind Linda that she does not have to disclose to these people the reasons for her need for support, but can simply ask if they would be willing to take on specific tasks (e.g., care for her children for an afternoon while she visits the doctor).
  - Follow up with Linda to find out if these recommendations were helpful and whether she may require additional care.

11
Women's Stories of Recovery

Roxanne's Story

I had ignored the early warning signs in my relationship with my boyfriend because I believed being with someone—anyone—was better than having no one, especially at the age of 29. I had always wanted to have a partner. And I also desperately wanted a child. I had what I call "the mother gene"—the desire from early on to be a mother.

So when I accidentally became pregnant a couple of months into our relationship, I was determined to keep the child. But I was scared. I didn't want my child to grow up without both parents, as I had.

I was raised by my grandparents from the age of seven months, although my mother and her husband raised my brother. Though my family is Guyanese, I was born in Ottawa. I didn't learn about my real father until I was five years old. I later found out that my father has about 12 children from six different women.

As you can imagine, I grew up feeling rejected by my parents and displaced at having to live with my grandparents. I didn't want my daughter to also grow up without a parent. So I tried to make my relationship with my boyfriend work. Three months before the delivery, I moved in with him, and a low-grade depression crept in. My boyfriend constantly put me down, and forbid me from talking to any of my male friends or doing things I did before we met, like travelling. He became very suspicious of me, and said he doubted that the baby was his. Slowly, I lost myself and began transforming into what he wanted.

After giving birth to my daughter, I called a friend from the hospital crying. My hormones were all out of whack. I felt stressed at the idea of relinquishing what little power I believed I had left over my life—in terms of my career and aspirations. I was faced with the reality that if things didn't work out, I was going to be all alone. Becoming a single parent hadn't been one of my goals. As a first generation Canadian and woman of colour, I understood the importance of lightening the burden for subsequent generations: I wanted to be able to offer a child a solid foundation with financial security, and a good education. I was pretty sure I could not do this with my current boyfriend.

My daughter's birth was an intensive lesson in parental accountability. While I loved her, I was struggling as a new mother. My boyfriend never helped out. Neither my mother nor other family were around. And I didn't have friends with babies, so I was really isolated. Everything in my life was baby-related or involved domesticity. If I left the apartment to take my daughter for a walk, my boyfriend would accuse me of parading our child around the streets.

From the time my daughter was born, my boyfriend was becoming more and more abusive. He would leave for work early in the morning, come in late and then expect dinner. He would throw things at me, and had started withdrawing money from my bank account for what I suspected was a drug problem.

I knew I had to stabilize my mental health for the sake of my daughter. I thought painting a section of our basement apartment bright yellow would lift my spirits and energy level, and make the place feel less dark. But my depression continued. I lost interest in my appearance and would sometimes go days without showering. My boyfriend didn't seem to notice or care. If he did, he never said anything.

One good day, I got myself and my daughter ready, and we paid a visit to the doctor who delivered her. As we were leaving the hospital, I noticed a bunch of yellow brochures with a daisy on the front cover, spread out on the counter in a washroom. They had information about shelters and what to do if you thought you were being abused. Of course, I didn't want to admit this was happening to me, but knew the abuse was escalating.

Somehow, I found the strength to call one of the shelters for abused women and children to inquire about how it worked, and two days before my daughter's first birthday we fled our apartment, leaving behind her biological father. We sought refuge at the shelter for three months.

During our time there, my family doctor referred me to a brilliant psychiatrist who helped me understand why I had stayed in yet another toxic relationship. The people I know from Caribbean and Latin American communities don't seek treatment and ignore mental health issues because of the negative connotations associated with consulting a psychiatrist or psychotherapist. No one wants to be stigmatized as their "head ain't good." And many rationalize that God will take care of the problem. While I too had concerns about speaking to a therapist—I didn't want to be considered crazy or a bad mother—I knew that I had to do something to help myself.

After working a short time with my psychiatrist, I realized that leaving my boyfriend was my healthiest alternative. The decision eventually gave both my daughter and I an invaluable gift—peace of mind. My psychiatrist asked me if I felt I needed to take medication to alleviate the depression, but I didn't want to go that route. I looked into natural remedies and found some herbal drops that seemed to balance my hormones. The belief in myself and the belief that God put me here to make a valuable contribution to society kept me going. Being my daughter's role model also gave me the strength and will to live. While in the shelter, I began writing and volunteer-producing again for a community television station. Resuming what I had been doing before being overcome by depression helped take my mind off the negativity.

I knew that I wasn't the first woman to experience disappointment of this magnitude, and I wouldn't be the last. But I didn't want to become another statistic. During my stay in the shelter, I saw women from various ethnic groups who had encountered abuse and depression. I wanted to succeed by overcoming my issues to help not only myself but others who might find themselves in a similar situation. To do this, I have had to set standards about how I want to live where none ever existed. My role as a parent means continuing to strive to be the best I can be: a genuine example for my daughter.

Today, I am no longer depressed, and try to maintain a healthy outlook toward life with artistic and academic pursuits.

Sheri's Story

I generally go through life trying to be an optimist. When the bad days come, I assume that there must be a lesson to be learned. People often comment about how happy I seem. They say, "Whenever I talk to you, things seem to be a little bit brighter."

These same people would be shocked to know that I've had postpartum depression (PPD). I've actually had PPD three times, once with each of my daughters, who are now three, nine and 10 years old. I've coped with these bouts of depression in between doing a B.Sc. in biology, graduating from a medical laboratory technologist program and working as a laboratory technologist.

My first experience with PPD was the worst. I had no idea what was happening to me. I suffered from insomnia, despair, uncontrollable crying, obsessive-compulsive behaviour and a lack of appetite.

At the beginning, my daughter's cranky period would last from 6 pm until 1 am. As she got older, the cranky times didn't last as long, so I would do the dishes and tidy up before going to bed. Then, when it was time to sleep, I would lie in bed reviewing a list in my head: do the laundry, iron the clothes, take something out of the freezer for supper, repair those pants.... The list goes on and on, and the fear is always the same: if I don't get it done, my world will fall apart. By 4:30 a.m., it's time to feed the baby again and I've only been asleep for two hours. But I can't wake my husband up as he has to work during the day. So I get up and feed the baby, and put her back to sleep. It's now 5:30 a.m. and the list begins again. Finally, at around 6:30 a.m., I fall asleep until 8:00 a.m. Then the day begins again.

I'm tired but I have to get my list done. If things don't go the way I want them to (which rarely happens when you have kids), I lose it and get very angry. Then I feel guilty. How can I be such a horrible person and be so angry for such a little thing? So then I cry and feel like I should just run away. I just don't like the way things are going. Nobody seems to love me or want to help me. Then everything seems to calm down for a while, and I'm happy again getting back to my list. This is the cycle that repeats itself about four or five times a day.

I tell my husband that no one seems to care. He says that I should get some help. Then one day, when my daughter is about three months old, I start yelling at my husband for putting the TV remote down two inches from where I thought it should be. That's when alarms started going off.

A month later, when I was at the doctor for my daughter's four-month appointment, I asked about PPD. The doctor asked me a few questions and then handed me some samples of an antidepressant. After a couple of weeks, the medication worked great. I slept well. I was my fun-loving self again, and I was enjoying my new daughter and her tiny accomplishments.

Then, on a follow-up visit with my family doctor, I was told (erroneously, as I was later to discover) that I could not take the antidepressant while I was breastfeeding. That started a rollercoaster of different drugs until finally, with the advice of Motherisk, I was told I could go back on the original drug I had been taking. I stayed on the drug until my daughter was 12 months old and then slowly weaned myself off. During this time, I also formed an informal support network with other mothers from a local play group. We discovered that many of us had had similar experiences with PPD, which created a bond between us. We continue to meet today.

When I became pregnant a second time, I wondered if I would suffer from PPD again. I decided that if a second episode were to occur, this time I would be prepared. I would try all drug free avenues first. I would take care of myself: sleep, exercise, and get out of the house as much as possible.

But my second pregnancy turned out to be very stressful. Both of my grandmothers passed away and my husband's cousin drowned after an ice fishing accident. The stress took its toll. I went into premature labour at 35 weeks. The labour then stopped, but a follow-up ultrasound revealed that the umbilical cord was wrapped around the baby's neck several times. After much deliberation, I decided to opt for a scheduled Caesarean to ensure an expected arrival with people available to take care of my baby should anything go wrong.

My second daughter arrived quite healthy, despite a few bruises left from the cord around her neck. Then on day three—the dreaded Baby Blue Day—I woke up feeling like my heart was pounding out of my chest. I couldn't breathe, and I was quivering uncontrollably. I convinced the nurse to take the baby to the nursery because I could not take care of her in this kind of shape. I called my husband but he couldn't come right away because he had to take care of our older daughter. It wasn't until a few years later that I realized that I had had a panic attack.

After the panic attack, I took things easy to try and recover from surgery. But a few weeks later, the cycle started again—the insomnia, the rise in irritability, the outbursts, the crying and despair. I tried to cope by getting out of the house— taking the kids for walks, going to the playground—but this only helped marginally. After three weeks, I went back to the doctor and got another prescription for the antidepressant I had been on before. After two weeks, I was back to my normal self again, enjoying the mad chaos of motherhood.

In my third pregnancy, I started feeling bouts of depression when I was six weeks pregnant. Initially, I tried to ignore the symptoms, not realizing that the depression could start during pregnancy. When I was about five months pregnant, I began taking herbal remedies. I then switched to an antidepressant about three weeks after my third daughter was born.

Because my third daughter was born in December, while my other two daughters were in school, I could rest during the day while she slept. Things went well until the beginning of summer. At first, I truly enjoyed having all three at home. There were many of what I call "memory pictures" (moments I freeze in my mind). Then all of a sudden, I started to feel myself slip again. The doctor then increased my dose until I returned to work. Since then, I have switched to another antidepressant because I had side-effects from the first one. I still feel anxious from time to time, but I now have coping mechanisms to deal with the anxiety.

These are my different experiences with PPD. If there is anything that could have helped me along the way, it would have been to educate myself and the people I was in contact with about PPD. Everyone who works with new mothers need to know about PPD—the medical profession (nurses and doctors), midwives, doulas and early childhood educators. We live in a fast-paced society, but we must slow down for the welfare of our children and families. With proper education about PPD, we can prevent suffering. With proper understanding, depression in new mothers can be recognized and treated.

By speaking out about PPD, I am hoping to play a role in making people informed.

References

Abramowitz, J.S., Schwartz, S.A. & Moore, K.M. (2003). Obsessional thoughts in postpartum females and their partners: Content, severity and relationship with depression. *Journal of Clinical Psychology in Medical Settings, 10,* 157–164.

Addiction Research Foundation (Centre for Addiction and Mental Health) (1996). *The Hidden Majority: A Guidebook on Alcohol and Other Drug Issues for Counsellors Who Work with Women.* Toronto: author.

Ahokas, A., Kaukoranta, J., Wahlbeck, K. & Aito, M. (2001). Estrogen deficiency in severe postpartum depression: Successful treatment with sublingual physiologic 17beta-estradiol: A preliminary study. *Journal of Clinical Psychiatry, 62*(5), 332–336.

Altshuler, L.L., Cohen, L.S., Moline, M.L., Kahn, D.A., Carpenter, D. & Docherty, J.P. (2001). The expert consensus guideline series: Treatment of depression in women. *Postgraduate Medical Journal, March,* 1–107.

Amato, P.R. (1993). Urban-rural differences in helping friends and family members. *Social Psychology Quarterly, 56,* 249–262.

American Academy of Pediatrics Committee on Drugs (2001). The transfer of drugs and other chemicals into human milk. *Pediatrics, 108*(3), 776–789.

American Psychiatric Association. (1994). *Diagnostic and Statistical Manual of Mental Disorders (4th ed.).* Washington, DC: author.

Appleby, L., Koren, G. & Sharp, D. (1999). Depression in pregnant and postnatal women: An evidence-based approach to treatment in primary care. *British Journal of General Practice, 49,* 780–782.

Appleby, L., Warner, R., Whitton, A. & Faragher, B. (1997). A controlled study of fluoxetine and cognitive behavioural counselling in the treatment of postnatal depression. *British Medical Journal, 314*(7085), 932–936.

Areias, M.E.G., Kumar, R., Barros, H. & Figueiredo, E. (1996). Correlates of postnatal depression in mothers and fathers. *British Journal of Psychiatry, 196*(1), 36–41.

Arendt, M. & Elklit, A. (2001). Effectiveness of psychological debriefing. *Acta Psychiatrica Scandinavica, 104*(6), 423–437.

Armstrong, K.L., Fraser, J.A., Dadds, M.R. & Morris, J. (1999). A randomized, controlled trial of nurse home visiting to vulnerable families with newborns. *Journal of Paediatrics & Child Health, 35*(3), 237–244.

Armstrong, K.L., Fraser, J.A., Dadds, M.R. & Morris, J. (2000). Promoting secure attachment, maternal mood and child health in a vulnerable population: A randomized controlled trial. *Journal of Paediatrics & Child Health, 36*(6), 555–562.

Astbury, J., Brown, S., Lumley, J. & Small, R. (1994). Birth events, birth experiences and social differences in postnatal depression. *Australian & New Zealand Journal of Public Health, 18*, 176–184.

Austin, M. & Lumley, J. (2003). Antenatal screening for postnatal depression: A systematic review. *Acta Psychiatrica Scandinavica, 107*(1), 10–17.

Barbara, A. & Doctor, F. (2004). *Asking the Right Questions 2: Talking with Clients about Sexual Orientation and Gender Identity in Mental Health, Counselling and Addiction Settings.* Toronto: Centre for Addiction and Mental Health.

Barclay, L. & Kent, D. (1998). Recent immigration and the misery of motherhood: A discussion of pertinent issues. *Midwifery, 14*, 4–9.

Beck, C. T. (1993). Teetering on the edge: A substantive theory of postpartum depression. *Nursing Research, 42*(1), 42–48.

Beck, C. T. (1996). A meta-analysis of predictors of postpartum depression. *Nursing Research, 45*, 297–303.

Beck, C.T. (2001). Predictors of postpartum depression: An update. *Nursing Research, 50*, 275–285.

Beck, C.T. & Gable, R.K. (2000). Postpartum Depression Screening Scale: Development and psychometric testing. *Nursing Research, 49*(5), 272–282.

Beck, C.T. & Gable, R.K. (2001a). Comparative analysis of the performance of the Postpartum Depression Screening Scale with two other depression instruments. *Nursing Research, 50*(4), 242–250.

Beck, C.T. & Gable, R.K. (2001b). Further validation of the Postpartum Depression Screening Scale. *Nursing Research, 50*(3), 155–164.

Bennett, H.A., Einarson, A., Taddio, A., Koren, G. & Einarson, T.R. (2004). Prevalence of depression during pregnancy: Systematic review. *Obstetrics & Gynecology, 103*(4), 698–709.

Bloch, M., Schmidt, P.J., Danaceau, M., Murphy, J., Nieman, L., & Rubinow, D.R. (2000). Effects of gonadal steroids in women with a history of postpartum depression. *American Journal of Psychiatry, 157*, 924–930.

Boyce, P.M. & Todd, A.L. (1992). Increased risk of postnatal depression after emergency caesarean section. *Medical Journal of Australia, 157*, 172–174.

Bradley, K.A., Boyd-Wickizer, J., Powell, S.H. & Burman, M.L. (1998). Alcohol screening questionnaires in women: A critical review. *Journal of the American Medical Association, 280*, 166–171.

Brennan, P.A., Le Brocque, R. & Hammen, C. (2003). Maternal depression, parent-child relationships, and resilient outcomes in adolescence. *Journal of the American Academy of Child & Adolescent Psychiatry, 42,* 1469–1477.

Brockington, I.F. & Cox-Roper, A. (1988). The nosology of puerperal mental illness. In I.F. Brockington & R. Kumar (Eds.), *Motherhood and Mental Illness 2: Causes and Consequences* (pp. 86–97). London: Wright.

Brown, S. & Lumley, J. (2000). Physical health problems after childbirth and maternal depression at six to seven months postpartum. *British Journal of Obstetrics & Gynaecology, 107*(10), 1194–1201.

Brugha, T.S., Wheatley, S., Taub, N.A., Culverwell, A., Friedman, T., Kirwan, P., Jones, D.R. & Shapiro, D.A. (2000). Pragmatic randomized trial of antenatal intervention to prevent post-natal depression by reducing psychosocial risk factors. *Psychological Medicine, 30*(6), 1273–1281.

Buist, A. & Janson, H. (2001). Childhood sexual abuse, parenting and postpartum depression—a 3-year follow-up study. *Child Abuse & Neglect, 25,* 909–921.

Buist, A., Westley, D. & Hill, C. (1999). Antenatal prevention of postnatal depression. *Archives of Women's Mental Health, 1,* 167–173.

Cadman, D., Chambers, L., Feldman, W. & Sackett, D. (1984). Assessing the effectiveness of community screening programs. *Journal of the American Medical Association, 251*(12), 1580–1585.

Callahan, C.M., Dittus, R.S. & Tierney, W.M. (1996). Primary care physicians' medical decision making for late-life depression. *Journal of General Internal Medicine, 11*(4), 218–225.

Callahan, C.M., Hendrie, H.C., Dittus, R.S., Brater, D.C., Hui, S.L. & Tierney, W.M. (1994). Improving treatment of late life depression in primary care: A randomized clinical trial. *Journal of the American Geriatric Society, 42*(8), 839–846.

Chaaya, M., Campbell, O.M., El Kak, F., Shaar, D., Harb, H. & Kaddour, A. (2002). Postpartum depression: Prevalence and determinants in Lebanon. *Archives of Women's Mental Health, 5,* 65–72.

Chabrol, H., Teissedre, F., Armitage, J., Danel, M. & Walburg, V. (2004). Acceptability of psychotherapy and antidepressants for postnatal depression among newly delivered mothers. *Journal of Reproductive & Infant Psychology, 22*(1), 5–12.

Chabrol, H., Teissedre, F., Saint-Jean, M., Teisseyre, N., Roge, B. & Mullet, E. (2002). Prevention and treatment of post-partum depression: A controlled randomized study on women at risk. *Psychological Medicine, 32*(6), 1039–1047.

Chen, C.H., Wu, H.Y., Tseng, Y.F., Chou, F.H. & Wang, S.Y. (1999). Psychosocial aspects of Taiwanese postpartum depression phenomenological approach: A preliminary report. *Kao-Hsiung i Hsueh Ko Hsueh Tsa Chih [Kaohsiung Journal of Medical Sciences], 15*(1), 44–51.

Cicchetti, D., Rogosch, F.A. & Toth, S.L. (1998). Maternal depressive disorder and contextual risk: Contributions to the development of attachment insecurity and behavior problems in toddlerhood. *Developmental Pscychopathology, 10*(2), 283–300.

Cooper P.J., Murray, L., Wilson, A. & Romaniuk, H. (2003). Controlled trial of the short- and long-term effect of psychological treatment of post-partum depression: I. Impact on maternal mood. *British Journal of Psychiatry, 182,* 412–419.

Cox, J. & Holden, J. (2003). *Perinatal Mental Health: A Guide to the Edinburgh Postnatal Depression Scale.* London: Gaskell.

Cox, J.L., Holden, J.M. & Sagovsky, R. (1987). Detection of postnatal depression. Development of the 10-item Edinburgh Postnatal Depression Scale. *British Journal of Psychiatry, 150,* 782–786.

Dalton, K. (1976). Progesterone or progestogens? *British Medical Journal, 2*(6046), 1257.

Dalton, K. (1994). Postnatal depression and prophylactic progesterone. *British Journal of Family Planning, 19*(Suppl.), 10–12.

Danaci, A.E., Dinc, G., Deveci, A., Sen, F.S. & Icelli, I. (2002). Postnatal depression in Turkey: Epidemiological and cultural aspects. *Social Psychiatry & Psychiatric Epidemiology, 37,* 125–129.

Dankner, R., Goldberg, R.P., Fisch, R.Z. & Crum, R.M. (2000). Cultural elements of postpartum depression: A study of 327 Jewish Jerusalem women. *Journal of Reproductive Medicine, 45,* 97–104.

Dean, C., Dean, N.R., White, A. & Liu, W.Z. (1995). An adoption study comparing the prevalence of psychiatric illness in women who have adoptive and natural children compared with women who have adoptive children only. *Journal of Affective Disorders, 34,* 55–60.

Dennis, C.L. (2003a). The effect of peer support on postpartum depression: A pilot randomized controlled trial. *Canadian Journal of Psychiatry, 48,* 115–124.

Dennis, C.L. (2003b). Peer support within a health care context: A concept analysis. *International Journal of Nursing Studies, 40*(3), 321–332.

Dennis, C.L. (2004a). Can we identify mothers at risk for postpartum depression in the immediate postpartum period using the Edinburgh Postnatal Depression Scale? *Journal of Affective Disorders, 78*(2), 163–169.

Dennis, C.L. (2004b). Preventing postpartum depression part I: A review of biological interventions. *Canadian Journal of Psychiatry, 49*(7), 467–475.

Dennis, C.L. (2004c). Preventing postpartum depression part II: A critical review of nonbiological interventions. *Canadian Journal of Psychiatry, 49*(8), 526–538.

Dennis, C.L. (2004d) Treatment of postpartum depression part 2: A critical review of non-biological interventions. *Journal of Clinical Psychiatry, 65,* 1252–1265.

Dennis, C.L. & Creedy, D. (2004). Psychosocial and psychological interventions for preventing postpartum depression. *The Cochrane Database of Systematic Reviews,* Issue 4.

Dennis, C.L., Janssen, P. & Singer, J. (2004). Identifying mothers at-risk for postpartum depression in the immediate postpartum period. *Acta Psychiatrica Scandinavica, 110,* 338–346.

Dennis, C.L. & Stewart, D. (2004). Treatment of postpartum depression part 1: A critical review of biological interventions. *Journal of Clinical Psychiatry, 65,* 1242–1251.

Dowrick, C. (1995). Does testing for depression influence diagnosis or management by general practitioners? *Family Practice, 12*(4), 461–465.

Dubovsky, S.L. & Buzan, R. (1999). Mood disorders. In R.E. Hales, S.C. Yudofsky & J.A. Talbott (Eds.), *Textbook of Psychiatry (3rd ed.)* (pp. 479–565). Washington, DC: American Psychiatric Press.

Eberhard-Gran, M., Eskild, A., Tambs, K., Samuelsen, S.O. & Opjordsmoen S. (2002). Depression in postpartum and non-postpartum women: Prevalence and risk factors. *Acta Psychiatrica Scandinavica, 106*(6): 426–433.

Elliott, S.A. & Leverton, T. (2000). Is the EPDS a magic wand? 2. Myths and the evidence base. *Journal of Reproductive and Infant Psychology, 18*(4), 297–307.

Elliott, S.A., Leverton, T.J., Sanjack, M., Turner, H., Cowmeadow, P., Hopkins, J. & Bushnell, D. (2000). Promoting mental health after childbirth: A controlled trial of primary prevention of postnatal depression. *British Journal of Clinical Psychology, 39*(Pt. 3), 223–241.

Epperson, C.N., Terman, M., Terman, J.S., Hanusa, B.H., Oren, D.A., Peindl, K.S. & Wisner K.L. (2004). Randomized clinical trial of bright light therapy for antepartum depression: Preliminary findings. *Journal of Clinical Psychiatry, 65*(3), 421–425.

Epstein, R. (2002). Lesbian families. In M. Lynn (Ed.), *Voices: Essays on Canadian Families* (pp. 76–102). Toronto: Nelson Canada.

Evins, G.G., Theofrastous, J.P. & Galvin, S.L. (2000). Postpartum depression: A comparison of screening and routine clinical evaluation. *American Journal of Obstetrics & Gynecology, 182*(5), 1080–1082.

Fergerson, S.S., Jamieson, D.J. & Lindsay, M. (2002). Diagnosing postpartum depression: Can we do better? *American Journal of Obstetrics & Gynecology, 186*(5), 899–902.

Forman, D.N., Videbech, P., Hedegaard, M., Salvig, J.D. & Secher, N.J. (2000). Postpartum depression: Identification of women at risk. *British Journal of Obstetrics & Gynaecology, 107*, 1210–1217.

Gage, J.D. & Kirk, R. (2002). First-time fathers: Perceptions of preparedness for fatherhood. *Canadian Journal of Nursing Research 34*(4), 15–24.

Gagnon, A.J., Tuck, J. & Barkun, L. (2004). A systematic review of questionnaires measuring the health of resettling refugee women. *Health Care for Women International, 25*, 111–149.

Gair, S. (1999). Distress and depression in new motherhood: Research with adoptive mothers highlights important contributing factors. *Child & Family Social Work, 4*, 55–66.

Gallo, J.J., Marino, S., Ford, D. & Anthony, J.C. (1995). Filters on the pathway to mental health care, II: Sociodemographic factors. *Psychological Medicine, 25*, 1149–1160.

Gibson, E. (1982). Homicide in England and Wales, 1967–1971. London: Pitman.

Glover, V., Liddle, P., Taylor, A., Adams, D. & Sandler, M. (1994). Mild hypomania (the highs) can be a feature of the first postpartum week. Association with later depression. *British Journal of Psychiatry, 164*(4), 517–521.

Goodman, J.H. (2004). Paternal postpartum depression, its relationship to maternal postpartum depression, and implications for family health. *Journal of Advanced Nursing, 45*, 26–35.

Goodman, S.H. & Gotlib, I.H. (1999). Risk for psychopathology in the children of depressed mothers: A developmental model for understanding mechanisms of transmission. *Psychological Review, 106*, 458–490.

Gopfert M., Webster, J. & Seeman, M.V. (2004). *Parental Psychiatric Disorder: Distressed Parents and Their Families (2nd ed.)*. Cambridge: Cambridge University Press.

Gordon, R. & Gordon, K. (1960). Social factors in prevention of postpartum emotional problems. *Obstetrics & Gynecology, 15*(4), 433–438.

Gorman, L.L. (2001). *Prevention of Postpartum Depression in a High Risk Sample.* Iowa City, IA: University of Iowa.

Grace, S.L. (2003). A review of Aboriginal women's physical and mental health status in Ontario. *Canadian Journal of Public Health, Revue Canadienne de Santé Publique, 94,* 173–175.

Gregoire, A.J., Kumar, R., Everitt, B., Henderson, A.F. & Studd, J.W. (1996). Transdermal oestrogen for treatment of severe postnatal depression. *Lancet, 347*(9006), 930–933.

Griepsma, J., Marcollo, J., Casey, C., Cherry, F., Vary, E. & Walton, V. (1994). The incidence of postnatal depression in a rural area and the needs of affected women. *Australian Journal of Advanced Nursing, 11,* 19–23.

Gunn, J., Lumley, J., Chondros, P. & Young, D. (1998). Does an early postnatal check-up improve maternal health: Results from a randomised trial in Australian general practice. *British Journal of Obstetrics & Gynaecology, 105*(9), 991–997.

Hammen, C. & Brennan, P.A. (2003). Severity, chronicity, and timing of maternal depression and risk for adolescent offspring diagnoses in a community sample. *Archives of General Psychiatry, 60,* 253–258.

Hannah, P., Adams, D., Lee, A., Glover, V. & Sandler, M. (1992). Links between early post-partum mood and post-natal depression. *British Journal of Psychiatry, 160,* 777–780.

Hapgood, C.C., Elkind, G.S. & Wright, J.J. (1988). Maternity blues: Phenomena and relationship to later post partum depression. *Australian & New Zealand Journal of Psychiatry, 22*(3), 299–306.

Harris, B., Fung, H., Johns, S., Kologlu, M., Bhatti, R., McGregor, A.M., et al. (1989). Transient post-partum thyroid dysfunction and postnatal depression. *Journal of Affective Disorders, 17*(3), 243–249.

Harris, B., Johns, S., Fung, H., Thomas, R., Walker, R., Read, G., et al. (1989). The hormonal environment of post-natal depression. *British Journal of Psychiatry, 154,* 660–667.

Harris, B., Lovett, L., Smith, J., Read, G., Walker, R. & Newcombe, R. (1996). Cardiff puerperal mood and hormone study. III. Postnatal depression at 5 to 6 weeks postpartum, and its hormonal correlates across the peripartum period. *British Journal of Psychiatry, 168*(6), 739–744.

Harris, B., Oretti, R., Lazarus, J., Parkes, A., John, R., Richards, C., et al. (2002). Randomised trial of thyroxine to prevent postnatal depression in thyroid-antibody-positive women. *British Journal of Psychiatry, 180,* 327–330.

Haskell, L. (2001). *Bridging Responses: A Front-Line Workers Guide to Supporting Women Who Have Post-Traumatic Stress.* Toronto: Centre for Addiction and Mental Health.

Hayes, B.A., Muller, R. & Bradley, B.S. (2001). Perinatal depression: A randomized controlled trial of an antenatal education intervention for primiparas. *Birth, 28*(1), 28–35.

Hendrick, V., Smith, L.M., Hwang, S., Altshuler, L.L. & Haynes, D. (2003). Weight gain in breastfed infants of mothers taking antidepressant medications. *Journal of Clinical Psychiatry, 64*(4), 410–412.

Heron, J., O'Connor, T., Evans, J., Golding, J., Glover, V. & the ALSPAC Study Team (2004). The course of anxiety and depression through pregnancy and the postpartum in a community sample. *Journal of Affective Disorders, 80,* 65–73.

Hiscock, H. & Wake, M. (2001). Infant sleep problems and postnatal depression: A community-based study. *Pediatrics, 107,* 1317–1322.

Hodnett, E.D., Lowe, N.K., Hannah, M.E., Willan, A.R., Stevens, B., Weston, J., et al. (2002). Effectiveness of nurses as providers of birth labor support in North American hospitals: A randomized controlled trial. *Journal of the American Medical Association, 288*(11), 1373–1381.

Holden, J. (1994). Using the Edinburgh Postnatal Depression Scale in clinical practice. In J. Cox & J. Holden (Eds.), *Perinatal Psychiatry: Use and Misuse of the Edinburgh Postnatal Depression Scale* (pp. 125–144). London: Gaskell.

Hollon, S.D. (1998). What is cognitive behavioural therapy and does it work? *Current Opinion in Neurobiology, 8*(2), 289–292.

Holroyd, E., Katie, F.K., Chun, L.S. & Ha, S.W. (1997). "Doing the Month": An exploration of postpartum practices in Chinese women. *Health Care for Women International, 18,* 301–313.

Huang, Y.C. & Mathers, N. (2001). Postnatal depression—biological or cultural? A comparative study of postnatal women in the UK and Taiwan. *Journal of Advanced Medical-Surgical Nursing, 33,* 279–287.

Hundt, C.L., Beckerleg, S., Kassem, F., Abu Jafar, A.M., Behnaker, I., Abu Saad, K., et al. (2000). Women's health custom made: Building on the 40 days postpartum for Arab women. *Health Care for Women International, 21,* 529–542.

Hyman, I. (2001). *Immigration and health.* Working Paper 01–05. Health Policy Working Paper Series. Ottawa: Health Canada. Available: www.hc-sc.gc.ca/iacb-dgiac/arad-draa/english/rmdd/wpapers/Immigration.pdf.

Jason J., Gilliland J.C. & Tyler C.W., Jr. (1983). Homicide as a cause of pediatric mortality in the United States. *Pediatrics, 72,* 191–197.

Johnstone, S.J., Boyce, P.M., Hickey, A.R., Morris-Yatees, A.D. & Harris, M.G. (2001). Obstetric risk factors for postnatal depression in urban and rural community samples. *Australian and New Zealand Journal of Psychiatry, 35,* 69–74.

Johnstone, A. & Goldberg, D. (1976). Psychiatric screening in general practice. A controlled trial. *Lancet, 1*(7960), 605–608.

Jones, I. & Craddock, N. (2001) Familiality of the puerperal trigger in bipolar disorder: Results of a family study. *American Journal of Psychiatry, 158*(6), 913–917.

Kaewsarn, P., Moyle, W. & Creedy, D. (2003). Traditional postpartum practices among Thai women. *Journal of Advanced Medical-Surgical Nursing, 41,* 358–366.

Karuppaswamy, J. & Vlies, R. (2003). The benefit of oestrogens and progestogens in postnatal depression. *Journal of Obstetrics and Gynaecology, 23*(4), 341–346.

Kelley, S.D.M., Sikka, A. & Venkatesan, S. (1997). A review of research on parental disability: Implications for research and counseling practice. *Rehabilitation Counseling Bulletin, 41,* 105–121.

Kelly, R.H., Zatzick, D.F. & Anders, T.F. (2001). The detection and treatment of psychiatric disorders and substance use among pregnant women cared for in obstetrics. *American Journal of Psychiatry, 158,* 213–219.

Kendell, R.E., Chalmers, J.C. & Platz, C. (1987). Epidemiology of puerperal psychoses. *British Journal of Psychiatry, 150*, 662–673.

Kit, L.K., Janet, G. & Jegasothy, R. (1997). Incidence of postnatal depression in Malaysian women. *Journal of Obstetrics and Gynaecology Research, 23*, 85–89.

Klerman, T.B. & Weissman, M.M. (1993). *New Applications of Interpersonal Psychotherapy*. Washington, DC: American Psychiatric Press Inc.

Laine, K., Heikkinen, T., Ekblad, U. & Kero P. (2003). Effects of exposure to selective serotonin reuptake inhibitors during pregnancy on serotonergic symptoms in newborns and cord blood monoamine and prolactin concentrations. *Archives of General Psychiatry, 60*, 720–726

Lane, A., Keville, R., Morris, M., Kinsella, A., Turner, M. & Barry, S. (1997). Postnatal depression and elation among mothers and their partners: Prevalence and predictors. *British Journal of Psychiatry, 171*, 550–555.

Lane, B., Roufeil, L.M., Williams, S. & Tweedie, R. (2001). It's just different in the country: Postnatal depression and group therapy in a rural setting. *Social Work in Health Care, 34*, 333–348.

Lavender, T. & Walkinshaw, S.A. (1998). Can midwives reduce postpartum psychological morbidity? A randomized trial. *Birth, 25*(4), 215–219.

Lawrie, T.A., Hofmeyr, G.J., De Jager, M., Berk, M., Paiker, J. & Viljoen, E. (1998). A double-blind randomised placebo controlled trial of postnatal norethisterone enanthate: The effect on postnatal depression and serum hormones. *British Journal of Obstetrics & Gynaecology, 105*(10), 1082–1090.

Lee, D.T., Yip, S.K., Chiu, H.F., Leung, T.Y., Chan, K.P., Chau, I.O., et al. (1998). Detecting postnatal depression in Chinese women: Validation of the Chinese version of the Edinburgh Postnatal Depression Scale. *British Journal of Psychiatry, 172*, 433–437.

Lee, D.T., Yip, A.S., Leung, T.Y. & Chung, T.K. (2000). Identifying women at risk of postnatal depression: Prospective longitudinal study. *Hong Kong Medical Journal, 6*, 349–354.

Levy-Shiff, R., Bar, O. & Har-Even, D. (1990). Psychological adjustment of adoptive parents-to-be. *American Journal of Orthopsychiatry, 60*, 258–267.

Linn, L.S. & Yager, J. (1980). The effect of screening, sensitization, and feedback on notation of depression. *Journal of Medical Genetics, 55*(11), 942–949.

Llewellyn, G. & McConnell, D. (2002). Mothers with learning difficulties and their support networks. *Journal of Intellectual Disability Research, 46*, 17–34.

Logsdon, M.C. (2004). Depression in adolescent girls: Screening and treatment strategies for primary care providers. *Journal of the American Medical Women's Association, 59*, 101–106.

MacArthur, C., Winter, H.R., Bick, D.E., Knowles, H., Lilford, R., Henderson, C., et al. (2002). Effects of redesigned community postnatal care on womens' health 4 months after birth: A cluster randomised controlled trial. *Lancet, 359*(9304), 378–385.

MacMillan, H.L., Walsh, C.A., Jamieson, E., Wong, M.Y., Faries, E.J., McCue, H., et al. (2003). The health of Ontario First Nations people: Results from the Ontario First Nations Regional Health Survey. *Canadian Journal of Public Health, 94*, 168–172.

Mao, Y., Moloughney, B.W., Semenciw, R.M. & Morrison, H.I. (1992). Indian Reserve and registered Indian mortality in Canada. *Canadian Journal of Public Health, 83*(5), 350–353.

Martinez-Schallmoser, L., Telleen, S. & MacMullen, N.J. (2003). The effect of social support and acculturation on postpartum depression in Mexican American women. *Journal of Transcultural Nursing, 14,* 329–338.

Matthey, S., Barnett, B., Howie, P. & Kavanagh, D.J. (2003). Diagnosing postpartum depression in mothers and fathers: Whatever happened to anxiety? *Journal of Affective Disorders, 74,* 139–147.

Matthey, S., Barnett, B., Kavanagh, D.J. & Howie, P. (2001). Validation of the Edinburgh Postnatal Depression Scale for men, and comparison of item endorsement with their partners. *Journal of Affective Disorders, 64,* 175–184.

Matthey, S., Barnett, B., Ungerer, J. & Waters, B. (2000). Paternal and maternal depressed mood during the transition to parenthood. *Journal of Affective Disorders, 60(2),* 75–85.

Matthey, S., Panasetis, P. & Barnett, B. (2002). Adherence to cultural practices following childbirth in migrant Chinese women and relation to postpartum mood. *Health Care for Women International, 23,* 567–575.

McIntosh, J. (1993). Postpartum depression: Women's help-seeking behaviour and perceptions of cause. *Journal of Advanced Nursing, 18(2),* 178–184.

McLennan, J.D. & Offord, D.R. (2002). Should postpartum depression be targeted to improve child mental health? *Journal of the American Academy of Child & Adolescent Psychiatry, 41(1),* 28–35.

McMahon, T.J., Winkel, J.D., Suchman, N.E. & Luthar, S.S. (2002). Drug dependence, parenting responsibilities, and treatment history: Why doesn't mom go for help? *Drug & Alcohol Dependence, 65,* 105–114.

Melges, F.T. (1968). Postpartum psychiatric syndromes. *Psychosomatic Medicine, 30,* 95–108.

Menaghann, E.G. (1990). Social stress and individual distress. *Research in Community and Mental Health, 6,* 107–141.

Meyer, I.H. (2003, May). *Minority stress and mental health in lesbians, gay men, and bisexuals.* Abstract presented at the American Psychiatric Association 156th Annual Meeting, San Francisco, California.

Misri, S., Kostaras, X., Fox, D. & Kostaras, D. (2000). The impact of partner support in the treatment of postpartum depression. *Canadian Journal of Psychiatry, 45,* 554–558.

Moran, N. (1996). Lesbian health care needs. *Canadian Family Physician, 42,* 879.

Morrell, C.J., Spiby, H., Stewart, P., Walters, S. & Morgan, A. (2000). Costs and effectiveness of community postnatal support workers: Randomised controlled trial. *British Medical Journal, 321(7261),* 593–598.

Mowbray, C.T., Oyserman, D., Zemencuk, J.K. & Ross, S.R. (1995). Motherhood for women with serious mental illness: Pregnancy, childbirth, and the postpartum period. *American Journal of Orthopsychiatry, 65,* 21–38.

Mrazek, P.J. & Haggerty, R.J. (1994). *Reducing risks for metal disorders—frontiers for prevention intervention research.* Washington, DC: National Academy Press.

Muir-Gray, J.A. (2001). *Evidence-Based Health Care: How to Make Health Policy and Management Decisions (2nd ed.).* London: Churchill Livingstone.

Murray, L. & Cooper, P.J. (1997). Postpartum depression and child development. *Psychological Medicine, 27(2),* 253–260.

Murray, L., Cooper, P.J., Wilson A. & Romaniuk H. (2003). Controlled trial of the short- and long-term effect of psychological treatment of post-partum depression: 2. Impact on the mother-child relationship and child outcome. *British Journal of Psychiatry, 182,* 420–427.

Murray, L., Hipwell, A., Hooper, R., Stein, A. & Cooper, P. (1996). The cognitive development of 5-year-old children of postnatally depressed mothers. *Journal of Child Psychology Psychiatry and Allied Disciplines, 37,* 927–935.

Nahas, V. & Amasheh, N. (1999). Culture care meanings and experiences of postpartum depression among Jordanian Australian women: A transcultural study. *Journal of Transcultural Nursing, 10,* 37–45.

Nahas, V.L., Hillege, S. & Amasheh, N. (1999). Postpartum depression: The lived experiences of Middle Eastern migrant women in Australia. *Journal of Nurse-Midwifery, 44*(1), 65–74.

Newport, J.D., Hostetter, A., Arnold, A. & Stowe, Z.N. (2002). The treatment of postpartum depression: Minimizing infant exposures. *Journal of Clinical Psychiatry, 63*(Suppl. 7), 31–44.

Nicholson, J., Sweeney, E.M. & Geller, J.L. (1998). Mothers with mental illness: I. The competing demands of parenting and living with mental illness. *Psychiatric Services, 49,* 635–642.

Nonacs, R. & Cohen, L.S. (1998). Postpartum mood disorders: Diagnosis and treatment guidelines. *Journal of Clinical Psychiatry, 59*(Suppl. 2), 34–40.

Oates, M.R., Cox, J.L. Neema, S., Asten P., Glangeaud-Freudenthal, N., Figueiredo, B., et al. (2004). Postnatal depression across countries and cultures: A qualitative study. *British Journal of Psychiatry—Supplementum, 184* (46), s10–16.

O'Hara, M.W. (1994). Postpartum depression: Identification and measurement in a cross-cultural context. In J. Cox & J. Holden (Eds.), *Perinatal Psychiatry: Use and Misuse of the Edinburgh Postnatal Depression Scale* (pp. 145–168). London: The Royal College of Psychiatrists.

O'Hara, M.W., Neunaber, D.J. & Zekoski, E.M. (1984). Prospective study of postpartum depression: Prevalence, course, and predictive factors. *Journal of Abnormal Psychology, 93,* 158–171.

O'Hara, M.W., Schlechte, J.A., Lewis, D.A. & Varner, M.W. (1991). Controlled prospective study of postpartum mood disorders: Psychological, environmental, and hormonal variables. *Journal of Abnormal Psychology, 100*(1), 63–73.

O'Hara, M.W. & Swain, A.M. (1996). Rates and risk of postpartum depression—a meta-analysis. *International Review of Psychiatry, 8,* 37–54.

Okano, T., Nagata, S., Hasegawa, M., Nomura, J. & Kumar, R. (1998). Effectiveness of antenatal education about postnatal depression: A comparison of two groups of Japanese mothers. *Journal of Mental Health, 7*(2), 191–198.

Paffenbarger, R.S. (1982). Epidemiological aspects of mental illness associated with childbearing. In I.F. Brockington & R. Kumar (Eds.), *Motherhood and Mental Illness* (pp. 21–36). London: Academic Press.

Pajulo, M., Savonlahti, E., Sourander, A., Ahlqvist, S., Helenius, H. & Piha, J. (2001). An early report on the mother-baby interactive capacity of substance-abusing mothers. *Journal of Substance Abuse Treatment, 20,* 143–151.

Pajulo, M., Savonlahti, E., Sourander, A., Helenius, H. & Piha, J. (2001). Antenatal depression, substance dependency and social support. *Journal of Affective Disorders, 65*(1), 9–17.

Patel, V., Rodrigues, M. & DeSouza, N. (2002). Gender, poverty, and postnatal depression: A study of mothers in Goa, India. *American Journal of Psychiatry, 159*, 43–47.

Peifer, K.L., Hu, T. & Vega, W. (2000). Help seeking by persons of Mexican origin with functional impairments. *Psychiatric Services, 51*, 1293–1298.

Pfost, K.S., Stevens, M.J. & Lum, C.U. (1990). The relationship of demographic variables, antepartum depression, and stress to postpartum depression. *Journal of Clinical Psychology, 46*, 588–592.

Pignone, M.P., Gaynes, B.N., Rushton, J.L., Burchell, C.M., Orleans, C.T., Mulrow, C.D., et al. (2002). Screening for depression in adults: A summary of the evidence for the U.S. Preventive Services Task Force. *Annals of Internal Medicine, 136*(10), 765–776.

Poole, N. & Isaac, B. (2001). *Apprehensions: Barriers to Treatment for Substance Using Mothers.* Vancouver, BC: British Columbia Centre of Excellence for Women's Health.

Pop, V.J., de Rooy, H.A., Vader, H.L., van der Heide, D., van Son, M.M. & Komproe, I.H. (1993). Microsomal antibodies during gestation in relation to postpartum thyroid dysfunction and depression. *Acta Endocrinologica (Copenh), 129*(1), 26–30.

Priest, S.R., Henderson, J., Evans, S.F. & Hagan, R. (2003). Stress debriefing after childbirth: A randomised controlled trial. *Medical Journal of Australia, 178*(11), 542–545.

Reading, J. (2003). The Canadian Institutes of Health Research, Institute of Aboriginal People's Health: A global model and national network for aboriginal health research excellence. *Canadian Journal of Public Health, Revue Canadienne de Santé Publique, 94*, 185–189.

Reid, M., Glazener, C., Murray, G.D. & Taylor, G.S. (2002). A two-centred pragmatic randomised controlled trial of two interventions of postnatal support. *British Journal of Obstetrics & Gynaecology, 109*(10), 1164–1170.

Reifler, D.R., Kessler, H.S., Bernhard, E.J., Leon, A.C. & Martin, G.J. (1996). Impact of screening for mental health concerns on health service utilization and functional status in primary care patients. *Archives of Internal Medicine, 156*(22), 2593–2599.

Renker, P.R. (1999). Physical abuse, social support, self-care, and pregnancy outcomes of older adolescents. *Journal of Obstetric, Gynecologic & Neonatal Nursing, 28*, 377–388.

Ritter, C., Hobfoll, S.E., Lavin, J., Cameron, R.P. & Hulsizer, M.R. (2000). Stress, psychosocial resources, and depressive symptomatology during pregnancy in low-income, inner-city women. *Health Psychology, 19*(6), 576–585.

Robinson, G.E. & Stewart, D.E. (2001). Postpartum disorders. In N. Stotland & D.E. Stewart (Eds.), *Psychological Aspects of Women's Health Care* (pp. 127–139). Washington, DC: American Psychiatric Press Inc.

Rodrigues, M., Patel, V., Jaswal, S. & de-Souza, N. (2003). Listening to mothers: Qualitative studies on motherhood and depression from Goa, India. *Social Science of Medicine, 57*, 1797–1806.

Romans-Clarkson, S.E., Walton, V.A., Herbison, G.P. & Mullen, P.E. (1990). Psychiatric morbidity among women in urban and rural New Zealand: Psycho-social correlates. *British Journal of Psychiatry, 156*, 84–91.

Ross, L.E., Gilbert Evans, S.E., Sellers, E.M. & Romach, M.K. (2003). Measurement issues in postpartum depression part 2: Assessment of somatic symptoms using the Hamilton Rating Scale for Depression. *Archives of Women's Mental Health, 6*(1), 59–64.

Ross, L.E., Gunasekera, S., Rowland, M., Steiner, M. (in press). Psychotropic medications in pregnancy. In A. Riecher-Rössler & M. Steiner (Eds.), *Perinatal Depression: From Bench to Bedside. Bibliotheca Psychiatrica, 172,* Basel, Switzerland: Karger.

Sackett, D.L. (1987). Screening in family practice: Prevention, levels of evidence, and the pitfalls of common sense. *Journal of Family Practice, 24*(3), 233–234.

Saisto, T., Salmela-Aro, K., Nurmi, J.E., Kononen, T. & Halmesmaki, E. (2001). A randomized controlled trial of intervention in fear of childbirth. *Obstetrics & Gynecology, 98*(5 Pt. 1), 820–826.

Schaper, A.M., Rooney, B.L., Kay, N.R. & Silva, P.D. (1994). Use of the Edinburgh Postnatal Depression Scale to identify postpartum depression in a clinical setting. *Journal of Reproductive Medicine, 39*(8), 620–624.

Seguin, L., Potvin, L., St. Denis, M. & Loiselle, J. (1999). Depressive symptoms in the late postpartum among low socioeconomic status women. *Birth, 26,* 157–163.

Serwint, J.R., Wilson, M.H., Duggan, A.K., Mellits, E.D., Baumgardner, R.A. & DeAngelis, C. (1991). Do postpartum nursery visits by the primary care provider make a difference? *Pediatrics, 88*(3), 444–449.

Shah, C.P. (1998). *Public Health and Preventive Medicine in Canada (4th ed.).* Toronto: University of Toronto Press.

Sharma, V. & Mazmanian, D. (2003). Sleep loss and postpartum psychosis. *Bipolar Disorder, 5*(2), 98–105.

Sharp, D., Hay, D.F., Pawlby, S., Schmucher, G., Allen, H. & Kumar, R. (1995). The impact of postnatal depression on boys' intellectual development. *Journal of Child Psychology & Psychiatry, 36*(8), 1315–1336.

Sheerin, F. (1998). Parents with learning disabilities: A review of the literature. *Journal of Advanced Nursing, 28,* 126–133.

Sichel, D.A., Cohen, L.S., Robertson, L.M., Ruttenberg, A. & Rosenbaum, J.F. (1995). Prophylactic estrogen in recurrent postpartum affective disorder. *Biological Psychiatry, 38*(12), 814–818.

Simon, G.E., VonKorff, M., Piccinelli, M., Fullerton, C. & Ormel, J. (1999). An international study of the relation between somatic symptoms and depression. *New England Journal of Medicine, 341,* 1329–1335.

Small, R., Brown, S., Lumley, J. & Astbury, J. (1994). Missing voices: What women say and do about depression after childbirth. *Journal of Reproductive & Infant Psychology, 12,* 19–22.

Small, R., Lumley, J., Donohue, L., Potter, A. & Waldenstrom, U. (2000). Randomised controlled trial of midwife led debriefing to reduce maternal depression after operative childbirth. *British Medical Journal, 321*(7268), 1043–1047.

Small, R., Lumley, J. & Yelland, J. (2003). How useful is the concept of somatization in cross-cultural studies of maternal depression? A contribution from the Mothers in a New Country (MINC) study. *Psychosomatic Obstetrics & Gynaecology, 24,* 45–52.

Spinelli, M.G. (2004). Maternal infanticide associated with mental illness: Prevention and the promise of saved lives. *American Journal of Psychiatry, 161*(9), 1548-1557.

Stamp, G.E., Williams, A.S. & Crowther, C.A. (1995). Evaluation of antenatal and postnatal support to overcome postnatal depression: A randomized, controlled trial. *Birth, 22*(3), 138–143.

Steinberg, S. (1996). Childbearing research: A transcultural review. *Social Science & Medicine, 43*, 1765–1784.

Steiner, M. (2002). Postnatal depression: A few simple questions. *Family Practice, 19*, 469–470.

Steiner, M. & Tam, W. (1999). Postpartum depression in relation to other psychiatric disorders. In L.J. Miller (Ed.), *Postpartum Mood Disorders* (pp. 47–63). Washington, DC: American Psychiatric Press, Inc.

Stern, G. & Kruckman, L. (1983). Multi-disciplinary perspectives on post-partum depression: An anthropological critique. *Social Science & Medicine, 17*, 1027–1041.

Stewart, D.E., (2000). Antidepressant drugs during pregnancy and lactation. *International Clinical Psychopharmacology, 15*(Suppl. 3), S19–S24.

Stewart, D.E. (1994). Incidence of postpartum abuse in women with a history of abuse during pregnancy. *Canadian Medical Association Journal, 151*, 1601–1604.

Stewart, D.E. & Cecutti, A. (1993). Physical abuse in pregnancy. *Canadian Medical Association Journal, 149*, 1257–1263.

Stewart, D.E., Robertson, E., Dennis, C.L., Grace, S.L. & Wallington, T. (2003, Oct.). *Postpartum Depression: Literature Review of Risk Factors and Interventions.* Toronto: Toronto Public Health.

Stuart, S. & O'Hara, M.W. (1995). Interpersonal psychotherapy for postpartum depression: A treatment program. *Journal of Psychotherapy Practice & Research, 4*(1), 18–29.

Teissedre, F. & Chabrol, H. (2004). Detecting women at risk for postnatal depression using the Edinburgh Postnatal Depression Scale at 2 to 3 days postpartum. *Canadian Journal of Psychiatry, 49*(1), 51–54.

Troutman, B.R. & Cutrona, C.E. (1990). Nonpsychotic postpartum depression among adolescent mothers. *Journal of Abnormal Psychology, 99*, 69–78.

Vanfraussen, K., Ponjaert-Kristoffersen, I. & Brewaeys, A. (2003). Family functioning in lesbian families created by donor insemination. *American Journal of Orthopsychiatry, 73*, 78–90.

Victoroff, V.M. (1952). Dynamics and management of para partum neuropathic reactions. *Diseases of the Nervous System, 13*, 291–298.

Warner, R., Appleby, L., Whitton, A. & Faragher, B. (1996). Demographic and obstetric risk factors for postnatal psychiatric morbidity. *British Journal of Psychiatry, 168*, 607–611.

Weier, K.M. & Beal, M.W. (2004). Complementary therapies as adjuncts in the treatment of postpartum depression. *Journal of Midwifery & Women's Health, 49*(2), 96–104.

Weissman, A.M., Levy, B.T., Hartz, A.J., Bentler, J., Donohue, M., Ellingrod, V.L. & Wisner, K.L. (2004). Pooled analysis of antidepressant levels in lactating mothers, breast milk and nursing infants. *American Journal of Psychiatry, 161*, 1066–1078.

Wells, K.B., Sherbourne, C., Schoenbaum, M., Duan, N., Meredith, L., Unutzer, J., Miranda, J., Carney, M.F. & Rubenstein, L.V. (2000). Impact of disseminating quality improvement programs for depression in managed primary care: A randomized controlled trial. *Journal of the American Medical Association, 283*(2), 212–220.

Wenzel, A., Haugen, E.N., Jackson, L.C. & Robinson, K. (2003). Prevalence of generalized anxiety at eight weeks postpartum. *Archives of Women's Mental Health, 6*, 43–49.

Whitton, A., Appleby, L. & Warner, R. (1996). Maternal thinking and the treatment of postnatal depression. *International Review of Psychiatry, 8*(1), 73–78.

Whooley, M.A., Stone, B. & Soghikian, K. (2000). Randomized trial of case-finding for depression in elderly primary care patients. *Journal of General Internal Medicine, 15*(5), 293–300.

Williams, J., Mulrow, C., Kroenke, K., Dhanda, R., Badgett, R., Omori, D. & Lee, S. (1999). Case-finding for depression in primary care: A randomized trial. *American Journal of Medicine, 106*(1), 36–43.

Wilson, J.M.G. & Junger, G. (1968). *Principles and practice of screening for disease.* Public Health Paper 34. Geneva: World Health Organization.

Wisner, K.L., Parry, B.L. & Piontek, C.M. (2002). Postpartum depression. *New England Journal of Medicine, 347*(3), 194–199.

Wisner, K.L., Perel, J.M., Peindl, K.S. & Hanusa, B.H. (2004). Timing of depression recurrence in the first year after birth. *Journal of Affective Disorders, 78*(3), 249–252.

Wisner, K.L., Perel, J.M., Peindl, K.S., Hanusa, B.H., Findling, R.L. & Rapport, D. (2001). Prevention of recurrent postpartum depression: A randomized clinical trial. *Journal of Clinical Psychiatry, 62*(2), 82–86.

World Health Organization. (2001). *The World Health Report 2001: Determinants of mental and behavioural disorders.* Retrieved November 26, 2004, from http://www.who.int/mental_health/en/.

Yamashita, H., Yoshida, K., Nakano, H. & Tashiro, N. (2000). Postnatal depression in Japanese women: Detecting the early onset of postnatal depression by closely monitoring the postpartum mood. *Journal of Affective Disorders, 58*(2), 145–154.

Yoshida, K., Marks, M.N., Kibe, N., Kumar, R., Nakano, H. & Tashiro, N. (1997). Postnatal depression in Japanese women who have given birth in England. *Journal of Affective Disorders, 43*(1), 69–77.

Yoshida, K., Yamashita, H., Ueda, M. & Tashiro, N. (2001). Postnatal depression in Japanese mothers and the reconsideration of "Satogaeri bunben." *Pediatric Nephrology, 43*, 189–193.

Zelkowitz, P. & Milet, T.H. (2001). The course of postpartum psychiatric disorders in women and their partners. *Journal of Nervous & Mental Disease, 189*, 575–582.

Zeskind, P.S. & Stephens, L.E. (2004). Maternal selective serotonin reuptake inhibitor use during pregnancy. *Pediatrics, 113*, 368–374.

Zlotnick, C., Johnson, S.L., Miller, I.W., Pearlstein, T. & Howard, M. (2001). Postpartum depression in women receiving public assistance: Pilot study of an interpersonal-therapy-oriented group intervention. *American Journal of Psychiatry, 158*(4), 638–640.

Zung, W.W. & King, R.E. (1983). Identification and treatment of masked depression in a general medical practice. *Journal of Clinical Psychiatry, 44*(10), 365–368.

Glossary

Aboriginal: the indigenous people of Canada and their descendants, including First Nations, Inuit and Metis peoples

Affective disorder: a mental condition involving mood and emotional problems

Anhedonia: persistent and pervasive loss of all pleasure and interest in activities usually enjoyed

Biopsychosocial model: a theoretical model that regards health, well-being and illness as resulting from the combined effects of biological, psychological and social factors

Bisexual: a person sexually attracted to and oriented toward both men and women, although not necessarily at the same time

Cognitive: describes the ability to think, reason, perceive and judge clearly and rationally

Cognitive-behavioural therapy (CBT): therapy aimed at improving coping skills by replacing distorted or negative thinking styles with more reality-based, logical and positive thought patterns

Control group: those taking part in a randomized controlled trial who do not receive the new treatment or strategy being evaluated. Researchers compare this group with another group (the intervention group) of similar individuals who do receive the new treatment to see if it is beneficial

Delusion: a fixed, unshakeable false belief with no rational or realistic basis, often held with conviction despite evidence of its unreality and cultural unacceptability

Doula: a support person (also called a monitrice or labour assistant); usually a woman knowledgeable about the normal course of childbirth who supports a woman (or couple) during labour and birth

Edinburgh Postnatal Depression Scale (EPDS): a 10-item self-report questionnaire developed specifically to detect postpartum depression (PPD)

Etiology: scientific assignment of the causes of a disease or condition

Family physician: a medically qualified doctor in general practice, with a two-year specialized residency (training) in family medicine

General practitioner: a medically qualified doctor in general practice

Hallucination: a perceptual distortion in which someone has a strong subjective perception of an object or event, not based on external reality or stimulus

Heterosexism: the assumption, overtly and/or covertly expressed, that all people are or should be heterosexual

Homophobia: irrational fear, hatred, prejudice or negative attitudes toward homosexuality and people who are gay or lesbian

Immigrant: a person who leaves his or her native country to settle in another country

Infanticide: killing an infant soon after birth

Interpersonal psychotherapy: a highly structured, brief form of psychotherapy that focuses on improving relationship roles, interpersonal dynamics and resolving conflicts

Intervention group: individuals taking part in a randomized controlled trial who receive the treatment or procedure being tested. Researchers compare the results in this intervention group with those from a similar group (the control group) that does not receive the new treatment to evaluate the effectiveness of the treatment

Lesbian: a female who is attracted to or whose primary sexual orientation is to other women, or who identifies herself as part of the lesbian community

Neuroticism: a term now seldom used in medical or clinical settings, referring to an overly worried and anxious manner of dealing with events, situations or relationships

Postpartum depression (PPD): depressive symptoms diagnosed soon after childbirth, usually within a year of delivery (often detectable within two to six weeks of the birth)

Postpartum Depression Screening Scale (PDSS): a recently developed 35-item self-report rating scale to detect postpartum depression in new mothers

Pre-eclampsia: development of hypertension (high blood pressure) during pregnancy

Prophylactic: an activity or treatment intended to prevent or slow down the course of a disease or illness

Prospective studies: studies that collect data and follow individuals before a disease or condition emerges

Psychiatrist: a doctor with a medical degree plus five years of specialized psychiatric training in diagnosing and treating mental health disorders

Psychologist: a non-medically qualified specialist in psychology, with the necessary training and licence to practise as a therapist, teach or do research

Psychosis: a severe mental health disorder typified by bizarre, disorganized or deranged behaviour and an inability to recognize reality or cope with everyday life

Puerperal/puerperium: the period immediately following childbirth

Randomized controlled trial: a study in which researchers randomly allocate individuals matched for age, gender and other characteristics (i.e., selected by chance) either to an intervention group (which receives the treatment being studied) or to a control group (not given the treatment). The aim is to determine whether or not the treatment or strategy being tested is effective or beneficial.

Refugee: a person who leaves his or her country of origin for fear of being persecuted on account of race, religion, political allegiance or some other identifiable characteristic

Self-care: the practice of looking after one's own health and well-being

Somatization: expression of anxiety or other emotional or mental symptoms as physical complaints

Stigmatization: social discrimination and ostracism, branding or marking a person (or making a person feel labelled) as "bad," inept or inferior

Stressor: any event, experience or environmental situation that produces mental, emotional or physical strain or tension and triggers the body's stress reaction

Suicidal ideation: persistent thoughts of self-harm, death or suicide; directly or indirectly expressed ideas of "being better off dead" or killing oneself

Appendix A

Edinburgh Postnatal Depression Scale

In the past seven days

1. I have been able to laugh and see the funny side of things:
❏ As much as I always could
❏ Not quite so much now
❏ Definitely not so much now
❏ Not at all

2. I have looked forward with enjoyment to things:
❏ As much as I ever did
❏ Rather less than I used to
❏ Definitely less than I used to
❏ Hardly at all

3. I have blamed myself unnecessarily when things went wrong:
❏ Yes, most of the time
❏ Yes, some of the time
❏ Not very often
❏ No, never

4. I have felt worried and anxious for no good reason:
❏ No, not at all
❏ Hardly ever
❏ Yes, sometimes
❏ Yes, very often

5. I have felt scared or panicky for no very good reason:
❏ Yes, quite a lot
❏ Yes, sometimes
❏ No, not very much
❏ No, not at all

6. Things have been getting on top of me:
❏ Yes, most of the time I haven't been able to cope at all
❏ Yes, sometimes I haven't been coping as well as usual
❏ No, most of the time I have coped quite well
❏ No, I have been coping as well as ever

7. I have been so unhappy that I have had difficulty sleeping:
❏ Yes, most of the time
❏ Yes, sometimes
❏ Not very often
❏ No, not at all

8. I have felt sad or miserable:
❏ Yes, most of the time
❏ Yes, quite often
❏ Not very often
❏ No, not at all

9. I have been so unhappy I have been crying:
❏ Yes, most of the time
❏ Yes, quite often
❏ Only occasionally
❏ No, never

10. The thought of harming myself has occurred to me:
❏ Yes, quite often
❏ Sometimes
❏ Hardly ever
❏ Never

Appendix B

Scoring the Edinburgh Postnatal Depression Scale

To score the EPDS, add up the scores associated with each response as indicated below. A woman scoring **10 or higher** should be referred to a physician or mental health specialist for further assessment. A score of **13 or higher** could indicate major depression.

In the past seven days

1. I have been able to laugh and see the funny side of things:
   - 0 As much as I always could
   - 1 Not quite so much now
   - 2 Definitely not so much now
   - 3 Not at all

2. I have looked forward with enjoyment to things:
   - 0 As much as I ever did
   - 1 Rather less than I used to
   - 2 Definitely less than I used to
   - 3 Hardly at all

3. I have blamed myself unnecessarily when things went wrong:
   - 3 Yes, most of the time
   - 2 Yes, some of the time
   - 1 Not very often
   - 0 No, never

4. I have felt worried and anxious for no good reason:
   - 0 No, not at all
   - 1 Hardly ever
   - 2 Yes, sometimes
   - 3 Yes, very often

5. I have felt scared or panicky for no very good reason:
   - 3 Yes, quite a lot
   - 2 Yes, sometimes
   - 1 No, not very much
   - 0 No, not at all

6. Things have been getting on top of me:
   - 3 Yes, most of the time I haven't been able to cope at all
   - 2 Yes, sometimes I haven't been coping as well as usual
   - 1 No, most of the time I have coped quite well
   - 0 No, I have been coping as well as ever

7. I have been so unhappy that I have had difficulty sleeping:
   3 Yes, most of the time
   2 Yes, sometimes
   1 Not very often
   0 No, not at all

8. I have felt sad or miserable:
   3 Yes, most of the time
   2 Yes, quite often
   1 Not very often
   0 No, not at all

9. I have been so unhappy I have been crying:
   3 Yes, most of the time
   2 Yes, quite often
   1 Only occasionally
   0 No, never

10. The thought of harming myself has occurred to me:
   3 Yes, quite often
   2 Sometimes
   1 Hardly ever
   0 Never

Cox, J.L., Holden, J.M. & Sagovsky, R. (1987). Detection of postnatal depression. Development of the 10-item Edinburgh Postnatal Depression Scale. *British Journal of Psychiatry, 150*, 782-786. Written permission must be obtained from the Royal College of Psychiatrists for copying and distribution to others or for republication (in print, online or by any other medium).

Translations of the scale, and guidance as to its use, may be found in Cox, J.L. & Holden, J. (2003). *Perinatal Mental Health: A Guide to the Edinburgh Postnatal Depression Scale.* London: Gaskell.

Appendix C

Antidepressant Dosages

Antidepressant Dosages Commonly Used*

* other dosages may be used under appropriate medical supervision

Class	Trade Name	Brand Name	Usual Start Dose (mg)	Usual Max Dose (mg)
SSRI	sertraline	Zoloft	25–50	200
	paroxetine	Paxil	10–20	60
	fluoxetine	Prozac	10–20	80
	citalopram	Celexa	10–20	60
	fluvoxamine	Luvox	25–50	300
SNRI	venlaxafine	Effexor	37.5	300
	duloxetine	Cymbalta	40	80
TCA	amitriptyline	Elavil	25	300
	desipramine	Norpramin	10–25	150
	imipramine	Tofranil	25	250
	nortriptyline	Aventyl	25	150
	doxepin	Sinequan	25	150
	trimipramine	Surmontil	25	200
	clomipramine	Anafranil	25	200

Appendix D

Resources for Service Providers and Parents

Educational Resources for Service Providers

Registered Nurses Association of Ontario (RNAO) Best Practice Guidelines for PPD
www.rnao.org/bestpractices

Registered Nurses Association of Ontario (2005). *Interventions for Postpartum Depression*. Toronto: Registered Nurses Association of Ontario.

The Marcé Society
www.marcesociety.com

An international society for research into the understanding, prevention and treatment of mental illness related to childbearing

Invest in Kids
www.investinkids.ca/Pages/Common/ContentPage.aspx

The latest research, strategies and best practices on parenting and early child development

Wellness: Health Care Information Resources (on pregnancy)
hsl.mcmaster.ca/tomflem/pregnan.html

Pregnancy links from *Health Care Information Resources*, McMaster University Health Sciences Library

Referral Sources for Service Providers

INFORMATION AND SUPPORT RELATED TO SUBSTANCE USE

R. Samuel McLaughlin Addiction and Mental Health Information Centre
1 800 463-6273

An initiative from the Centre for Addiction and Mental Health, which includes a toll-free information line, a telephone support line and resources on mental health and substance use problems for Ontarians

Addiction Clinical Consultation Service (ACCS)
1 888 720-ACCS (2227) or 416 595-6968

A program through the Centre for Addiction and Mental Health that provides consultation services to service providers who have clients with alcohol or other drug problems

Motherisk Information Line
416 813-6780

For information about the risk or safety of prescription and over-the-counter drugs, herbal products, chemicals, x-rays, chronic disease and infections during pregnancy and while breastfeeding

Motherisk Alcohol and Substance Use Helpline
1 877 327-4636

For information about the fetal effects of alcohol, nicotine and other substances, such as marijuana, cocaine and ecstasy

Is It Safe for My Baby?
www.camh.net/news_events/isitsafe_baby0603.html

Centre for Addiction and Mental Health (2003). *Is It Safe for My Baby?: Risks and Recommendations for the Use of Medication, Alcohol, Tobacco and Other Drugs During Pregnancy and Breastfeeding.* Toronto: author.

Pregnets
www.pregnets.org

A website aimed to help pregnant and postpartum women quit smoking

Women For Sobriety
www.womenforsobriety.org

Support and self-help for women with alcohol problems

CRISIS LINES AND SHELTERS

Hot Peach Pages
www.hotpeachpages.net/canada/index.html

An international list of agencies dealing with domestic violence

Shelternet
www.shelternet.ca

Canada-wide contact information for women's shelters and women's crisis lines organized by province, region and city/town

Centre for Suicide Prevention Website
www.suicideinfo.ca/csp/go.aspx?tabid=77

A Canada-wide listing of crisis centres and crisis lines organized by province

Parent Help Line
1 888 603-9100
www.parenthelpline.ca

A free, 24-hour telephone support and information line for parents

Kids Help Phone
1 800 668-6868
www.kidshelp.sympatico.ca

A free, 24-hour telephone support and information line for children and youth

Information for Parents

DIRECTORIES OF POSTPARTUM DEPRESSION SUPPORT GROUPS

Pacific Post Partum Support Society
www.postpartum.org/supportgroups.html

A listing of PPD support groups in Alberta, British Columbia, Quebec and Ontario

Our Sisters' Place
www.oursistersplace.ca/info/PDF/ppdsupportgroups.pdf

A listing of Ontario PPD support groups posted on the *Our Sisters' Place* website

SUPPORT FOR PREGNANT AND POSTPARTUM WOMEN

Canadian Association of Midwives
members.rogers.com/canadianmidwives/canada.html

Information on midwifery in the various Canadian provinces and territories

Canadian Doula Association
www.canadiandoulas.com

Information and support for expectant and new mothers. Includes information on how to find doulas and midwives, and questions to ask a birthing professional

La Leche League Canada Breastfeeding Support
www.lalecheleaguecanada.ca

Canadian chapter of La Leche International, providing information and contact numbers for breastfeeding support groups across Canada

Motherisk
www.motherisk.org

For information about the safety or risk of drugs, chemicals and disease during pregnancy and lactation

Dr. Newman's Pages on Breastfeeding
www.bflrc.com/newman/articles.htm

Close to 100 patient handouts and lectures by Dr. Jack Newman, Canadian breastfeeding expert

INFORMATION ON PPD AND OTHER POSTPARTUM MOOD DISTURBANCES

Women's Health Matters
www.womenshealthmatters.ca/centres/pregnancy/newborn/emotional_health.html

Canadian Mental Health Association
www.cmha.ca/english/info_centre/mh_pamphlets/mh_pamphlet_pp.htm

Depression After Delivery of Washington
www.ppmdsupport.com

Women's Health Concerns Clinic, St. Joseph's Healthcare Hamilton
www.stjosham.on.ca/whcc/perinatal.htm

Mood Disorders Society of Canada
www.mooddisorderscanada.ca/depression/ppd.htm

British Columbia Reproductive Mental Health Program
www.bcrmh.com/disorders/postpartum.htm

Postpartum Support International (PSI)
www.postpartum.net

Online PPD Support Group
www.ppdsupportpage.com

Women's Health Centre, St. Joseph's Health Centre
www.stjoe.on.ca 416 530-6850 (Toronto)
Calls returned to anywhere in Canada and the U.S.

Our Sisters' Place
www.oursistersplace.ca/osp.asp?mc=facts&aid=60

INFORMATION FOR FATHERS/PARTNERS

Boot Camp for New Dads
www.newdads.com

Practical advice for first-time dads

Dads Can
www.dadscan.ca

Promotes responsible and involved fathering

INFORMATION FOR DIVERSE FAMILIES

Canadian Adoption Support
www.familyhelper.net/arc/sup.html

A list of contacts for support agencies for adoptive parents

Family Pride Canada
familypride.uwo.ca

A national online resource centre for lesbian, gay, bisexual and trans parents

DisAbled Women's Network (DAWN) Canada
www.dawncanada.net/links.htm

An organization that addresses issues for women with disabilities

Index

O

Obstetric complications, 21
Ontario Psychiatric Outreach Program, 70
Our Sisters' Place, 94

P

Parenthood
chronic mental illness and, 103–105
marital conflict and, 20, 78, 124–125
PPD and mother-infant attachment, 83–84, 97
stressors and PPD, 81–82
Paroxetine (Paxil), 56
Partners. *See also* families; fathers
strategies for working with, 79–81, 124–125
developing parenting skills of, 113
developing support for PPD recovery, 79, 81–82
monitoring PPD symptoms, 62, 78–79
postpartum distress and, 82–83
role confusion, 81
role in child's development, 83
Paternal depression, 82–83
Paxil. *See* paroxetine
Peer support groups for mothers, 57–58, 112–113, 131
Physicians. *See* family physicians
Pinks, postpartum, 11
Postpartum depression (PPD). *See also*
depression; mood disorders; referrals; risk
factors; symptoms; treatments for PPD
causes of, 4–6
data collection issues, 19
impact of chronic or severe PPD on infant development, 83–84
mental illness in families and, 18–19
onset of, 4, 5
prevalence of, 4
recovery rates for, 35–36, 51
recurrences of, 6, 47, 48, 103–105, 130–132
Postpartum Depression Screening Scale (PDSS), 31–32
ethnocultural groups and, 90
Postpartum rituals and traditions of
ethnocultural groups, 90–91
Pregnancy
antenatal risk factors (Figure 2-1), 17
antidepressants and, 56
anxiety and, 18
depression and, 13, 18–20, 88
effectiveness of antenatal testing, 33

lack of social support and, 19–20
need for partner's support, 79
negative thinking styles and, 20
obstetric factors and PPD, 21
partner conflicts during, 20
physical abuse during, 97
prospective studies for PPD and, 16
screening for depression during, 33
stressful life events during, 19–20
substance use and depression during, 95
Prenatal. *See* antenatal; pregnancy; preventive interventions
Preventive interventions
antenatal and postnatal classes, 41
categories of, 40
continuity of care model, 43
early postpartum follow-up, 43–44
education and informational support, 43
effectiveness of, 49
flexible postpartum care, 44–45
hormonal interventions, 47–48
intrapartum support, 41
pharmacological interventions, 47
psychological interventions, 45–46
psychosocial interventions, 41–42
screening tests for diseases, 40
selecting types of, 49
Progesterone therapies, 48
Psychiatrists
emergency assessments and, 62, 64, 65
referral to, 71
role of, 13, 62, 72–73
Psychodynamic psychotherapy, 57
Psychological debriefing, 46
Psychologists and treatments, 45–46, 73
Psychomotor retardation or agitation, 8–9
Psychosis. *See also* suicidal ideation; chronic
mental illness and parenting
case study (Susan), 121–122
child care and, 103–105
mother's refusal of care, 68–69
hospital emergency department and, 70
psychiatrists and role of, 72–73
referrals for, 62–65
symptoms of, 12–13
Psychotherapies, 45–46, 57
Psychotherapists, 56–58, 74
Public health nurses, 74–75

Q

Questionnaires. *See* screening tools